Leading Authorities Pra
Sexually Transmitted Diseases

"Both sexes can use this guide to reach the proper diagnosis and management of these dangerous and potentially deadly conditions. An informative encyclopedia to reach for the next time you fear that STD has struck close to home."

—Niels H. Lauersen, M.D.
co-author, *It's Your Body: A Woman's Guide to Gynecology*

"This is one of the most timely and truly helpful books on health to have crossed my desk in recent years. . . . I hear story after story of women who are inadequately or improperly treated for what might have been trifling conditions, but which due to the ignorance of their doctors, are allowed to develop into major and chronic disorders. I only hope that so many patients will read this book that, in self-defense, doctors will have to read it too."

—Barbara Seaman
author of *The Doctors' Case Against the Pill* and *Women and the Crises in Sex Hormones*
Co-founder, National Women's Health Network

"*STD: A Commonsense Guide to Sexually Transmitted Diseases* is a rare find. Ms. Corsaro and Ms. Korzeniowsky are down-to-earth and nonjudgmental, they'll help you recognize trouble and meet it intelligently, and they talk in practical ways about VD *prevention*—perhaps the most important and least discussed public health issue associated with STD."

—Bruce Voeller, Ph.D.
former Director of the National Gay Task Force

". . . readable, authoritative, and in many ways, definitive . . . it's a relief that finally there is a resource to which interested people can turn."

—Samuel R. Knox
National Program Director
American Social Health Association

STD

A COMMONSENSE GUIDE TO SEXUALLY TRANSMITTED DISEASES

MARIA CORSARO &
CAROLE KORZENIOWSKY

FOREWORD BY JOSEPH A. SONNABEND, M.D.

An Owl Book

HOLT, RINEHART AND WINSTON
New York

Published by Holt, Rinehart and Winston,
383 Madison Avenue, New York, New York 10017.
Published simultaneously in Canada by Holt, Rinehart
and Winston of Canada, Limited.

Library of Congress Cataloging in Publication Data
Corsaro, Maria.
STD, a commonsense guide to sexually transmitted
diseases.
"An Owl book."
1. Venereal diseases. I. Korzeniowsky, Carole.
II. Title. III. Title: S.T.D., a commonsense guide
to sexually transmitted diseases.
RC200.2.C66 1982 616.95′1 81-7265 AACR2

ISBN: 0-03-059914-8

First published in hardcover by
St. Martin's Press, Inc. in 1980

First Owl Book Edition—1982

Illustrations by David Purnell

Printed in the United States of America
10 9 8 7 6 5 4 3 2 1

To our families and friends, whose love and support have been a constant inspiration.

ACKNOWLEDGMENTS

We'd like to thank three friends who got us started and helped to fuel our effort: Libby Finesmith, Waldemar Korzeniowsky and Joseph Sonnabend, our medical consultant.

Also, we'd like to express appreciation to professional colleagues who read parts or all of the manuscript and made invaluable suggestions: Dan William, M.D.; Carol Livoti, M.D.; Sharon Bromley, R.P.A.; John Kaim, M.D.; Marion Gold; and Esther Rome.

Contents

Foreword

SEXUALLY TRANSMITTED DISEASES are a reality for every person who is sexually active. They are an inevitable consequence of multiple partners. The difficulty in pointing this out is that it may be seen as a moralistic injunction against a more liberal approach to sexual behavior. This is not the case.

The potential effects of STDs may be devastating. Since it is likely that you do not have a personal physician to whom you can entrust your sexual well-being, it is imperative that you yourself take some responsibility. It is not only your own well-being, but also that of your community that is at stake.

This means that you should become aware of the degree of risk, the manifestations of these diseases, how they are diagnosed and treated, and what may be done to prevent their acquisition and to reduce their prevalence.

With respect to the diseases themselves, there are often inadequacies in the facilities that have traditionally been entrusted with their management. These include public health clinics, private physicians, hospital emergency rooms, and outpatient clinics. The best protection a sexually active individual can have is to be armed with some knowledge of the STDs.

In general, these diseases are well circumscribed and dealt with using standard procedures. These are relatively simple procedures and anyone can learn them. One of the benefits will be the ability to monitor the quality of care received. The authors have, in this book, presented information which will enable you to do just that.

No matter how excellent treatment is, it's hardly likely to make a substantial impact on the overall prevalence of STDs. Some degree of social responsibility is required. On a personal level, you should see that those whom you may have infected—or may have infected you—are taken care of. In this respect the assistance of a public health advisor should be welcomed rather than feared.

Preventive measures are discussed at some length in this book. Clearly the best way to deal with STDs is to take steps not to acquire them in the first place. It is a mistake to generalize about any of the measures advocated. For example, what may be suggested to an individual who makes contacts in a singles bar once or twice a week, may be entirely inappropriate for a married man who visits a gay bath house once or twice a year.

This book provides a guide for finding a suitable doctor in addition to giving you rational commonsense information on STDs. The least one should require from one's physician is medically sound treatment in a totally nonjudgmental setting as well as information regarding the care of sexual contacts.

If one swims in perilous waters, it helps to know the nature of the dangers. Look before you leap; if you still wish to proceed there is a good deal you can do to minimize the risk to yourself and to your partners.

—DR. JOSEPH A. SONNABEND

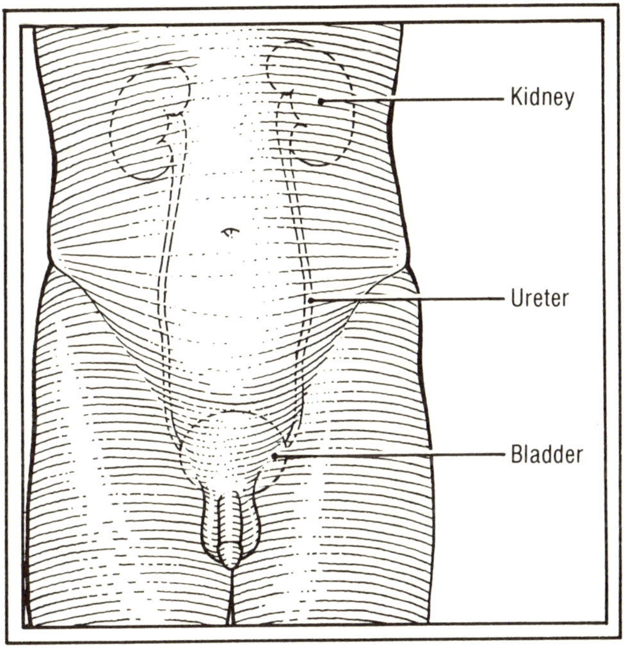

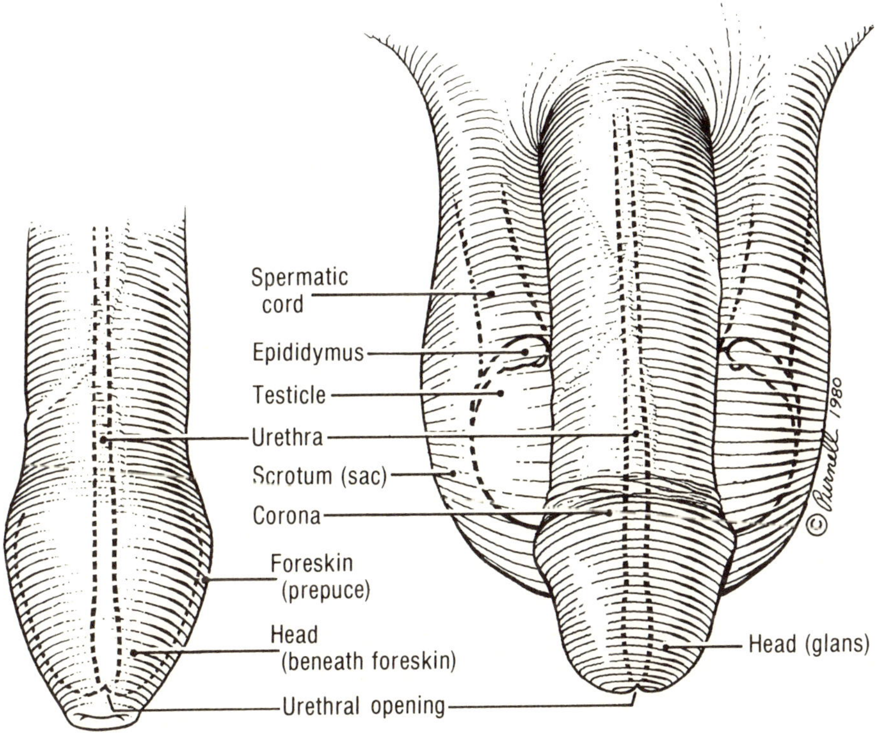

Uncircumcized

Circumcized

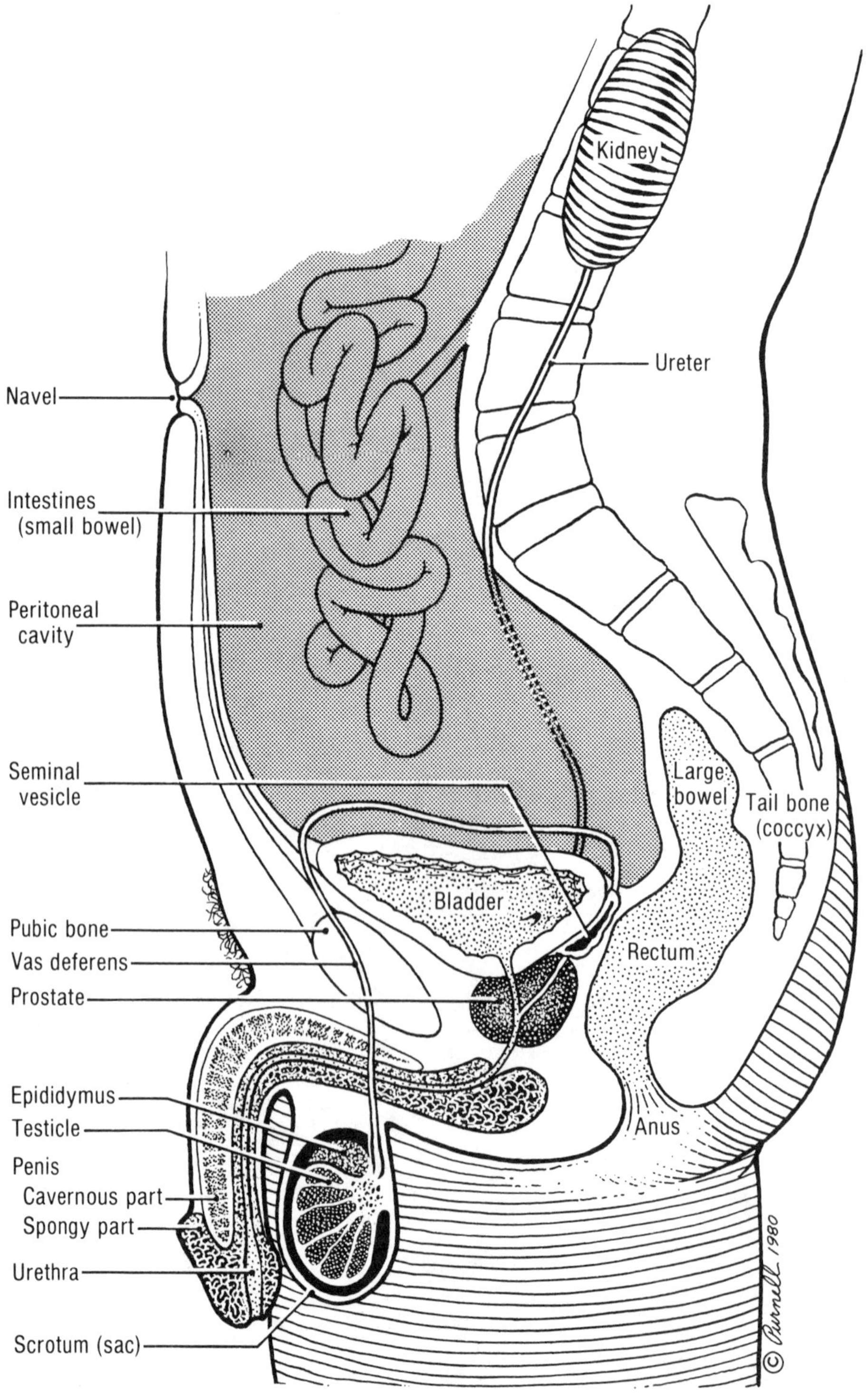

Kidney
Ureter
Navel
Intestines
(small bowel)
Peritoneal
cavity
Seminal
vesicle
Large
bowel
Tail bone
(coccyx)
Bladder
Pubic bone
Vas deferens
Rectum
Prostate
Epididymus
Anus
Testicle
Penis
Cavernous part
Spongy part
Urethra
Scrotum (sac)
© Purnell 1980

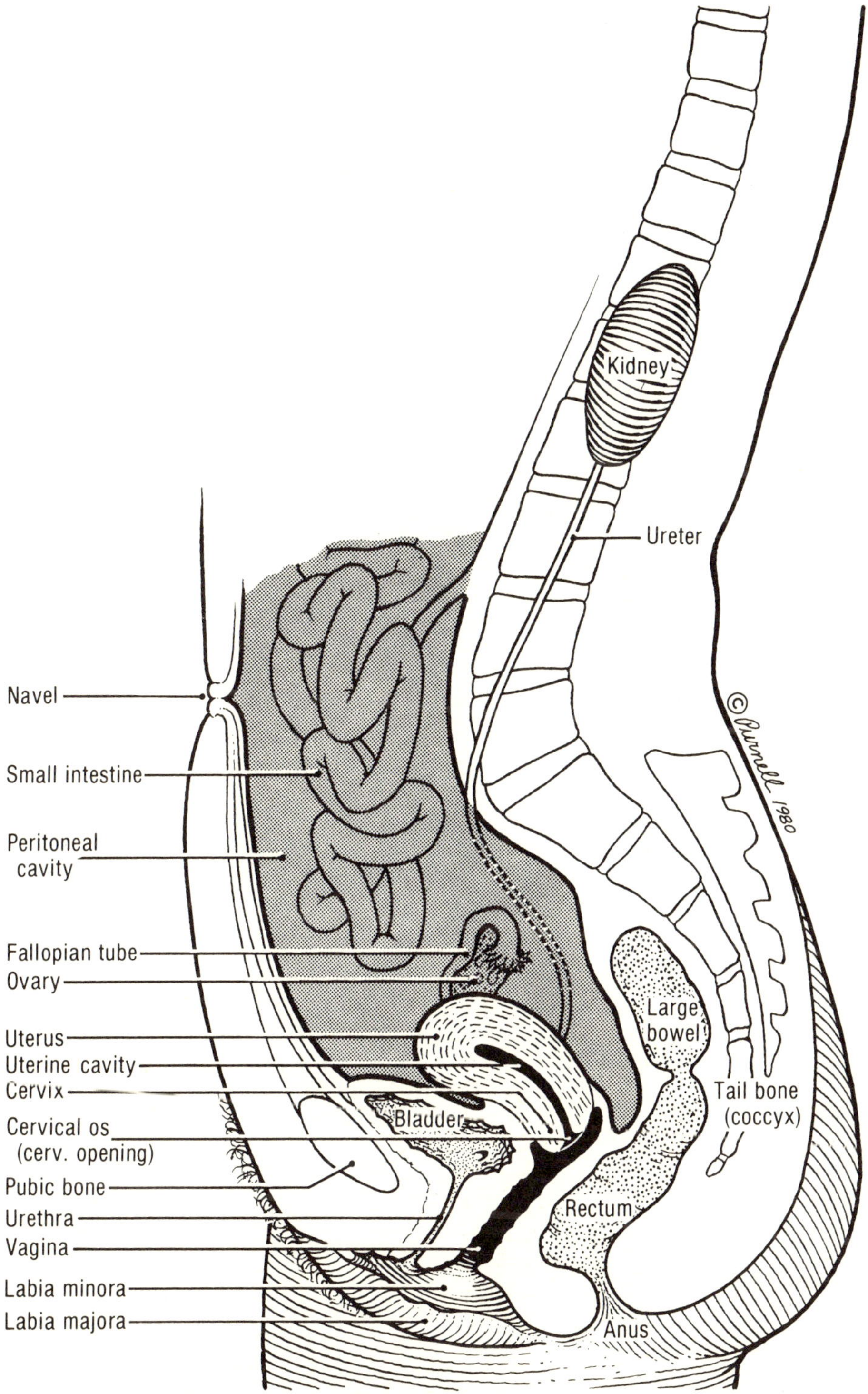
Navel
Small intestine
Peritoneal cavity
Fallopian tube
Ovary
Uterus
Uterine cavity
Cervix
Cervical os (cerv. opening)
Pubic bone
Urethra
Vagina
Labia minora
Labia majora
Kidney
Ureter
Large bowel
Bladder
Tail bone (coccyx)
Rectum
Anus
© Purnell 1980

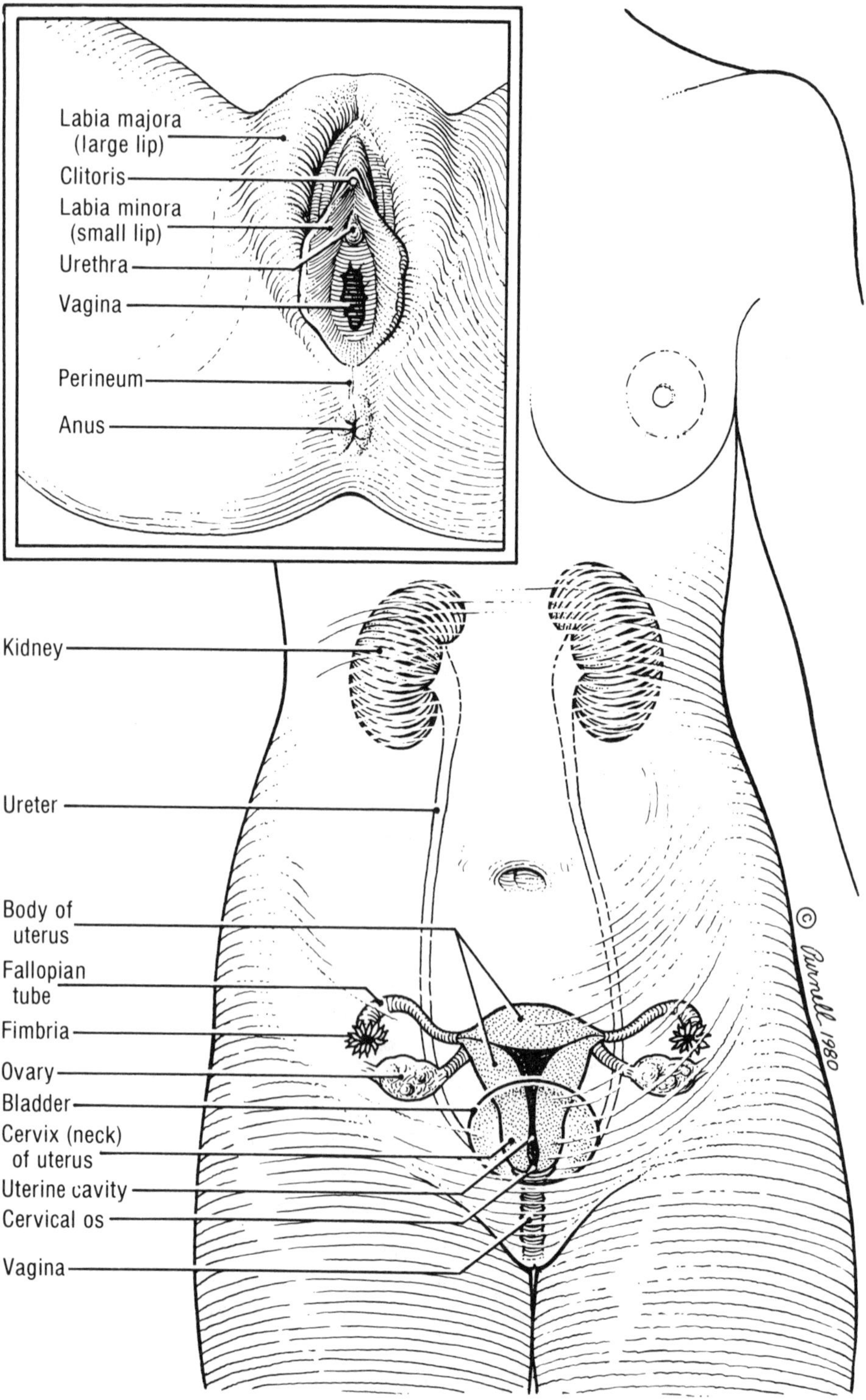
Labia majora (large lip)
Clitoris
Labia minora (small lip)
Urethra
Vagina
Perineum
Anus
Kidney
Ureter
Body of uterus
Fallopian tube
Fimbria
Ovary
Bladder
Cervix (neck) of uterus
Uterine cavity
Cervical os
Vagina
© Purnell 1980

Introduction: How to Use This Book

WE'RE ABOUT TO SAVE you time, money and worry. Worry, because sexually transmissible diseases (or STDs) are only a problem when they're not taken care of. And almost all of them can be taken care of easily. That is, they have sure-fire cures, something that can't be said yet about cancer, for example, or even the common cold.

Time and money, because people usually waste a lot of it unnecessarily, due to pure ignorance about STDs. Ignorance on the part of many doctors, as well as people in general. The first thing to realize is that there are an awful lot of STDs around, and that people are constantly giving them back and forth to each other like intimate little presents. As more people live freer lives, traveling between different partners and different places, the more likely we all are to contract an STD.

People have a hard time recognizing STDs. For various reasons:

—Although STDs are equal opportunity diseases, only certain of the links in an STD network may show the symptoms. So, if you feel fine, but your partner doesn't, you may have a closet case. Which should be taken care of, because (one) you may feel the effects later, and (two) you're spreading it.

—There are approximately twenty different STDs that have only one thing in common: they are usually transmitted sexually. So they have different symptoms and those symptoms can look like a lot of different diseases. You—or your doctor—have to be thinking about STDs as a possibility. Otherwise, you may end up wandering from doctor to doctor and even possibly to psychiatrists wondering what on earth is wrong with you.

—Because STDs are so intimately related to sex, lots of people are too embarrassed to be frank about them. That includes newspapers and magazines that refuse to advertise condoms although they are our most effective form of protection; doctors who don't want to "insult" their patients by asking the necessary questions; and patients who are also unwilling to ask questions because of a "what will they think of me" mentality.

Because STDs are on the rise, there is new information coming to light all the time. For some of the STDs, we are understanding better how they are transmitted among people; for others, we are developing newer and more effective medicines. It's not easy for a private physician, with all the other sicknesses s/he deals with, to keep abreast of the field of STDs. You can help your doctor and yourself by being prepared with some "intelligent guesses" about what you have, and an understanding of what is generally done about it.

Doctors diagnose disease by looking for physical symptoms, asking questions and doing proper testing. With

STDs, you can do a part of this. There are a number of symptoms—bumps, blisters, burning, etc.—that anyone can observe. Our book is designed to bring you from obvious symptoms to decisions about what to do for them. (Of course, you're free to read *STD* from cover to cover and we hope you do!)

The key on the next pages is your guide to the information you'll need if you suspect you've caught something from a sexual partner. If, for example, you have an itch, just look up itch in the key, locate the specific area of the itching and then turn to the suggested chapters (they're in alphabetical order). In each chapter, you'll find out how the disease is spread, what the symptoms are, what is usually done to cure it and/or relieve the symptoms, what else it might be * and anything else you should know to deal with your problem practically.

In some cases, we've addressed remarks directly to women, or gay males, or heterosexual males because they are at risk for a specific disease. We haven't done this for gay women since there is no evidence that they are at high risk for any of the STDs. Because children are often recipients of STDs through their close contact with parents, especially in childbirth, we've added notes to parents at the end of the chapters wherever applicable.

In front of the book are illustrations of the male and female reproductive systems with all of the relevant parts identified. Most people have never learned anatomy, but it is necessary to get a few of the terms and parts straight, if only for this reason: Doctors often expect you to know what they mean.

There's a glossary in the back of the book with short

* Where there's an asterisk after the name of a disease, it means we've handled it in detail in another section of the book.

descriptions of diagnostic tests, medicines and other words related to STDs but not in common usage. If any of the terms you encounter are unfamiliar, they're likely to be in the glossary.

Finally, we've added three appendixes filled with facts and helpful hints. Appendix A is reserved for women, wherein we explain the use of the speculum, an instrument which makes it possible for a woman to observe her own vagina and cervix. Changes in these two are important indications of several STDs in women.

Appendix B is an overview of your medical options. Will it be a private physician, a hospital out-patient department or a public health clinic? There are pros and cons to be considered for each of the situations.

Appendix C might, in fact, be the first section you will want to read. It is about prevention; how to have sex without STDs. If you can prevent STDs from happening, you won't have to worry about the rest of this book. And that would be the best nonuse of the book we can imagine.

The STD Key

IF YOU ARE MOST DISTRESSED BY:

1. A Burning Sensation
   During Urination: See herpes; gonorrhea; cystitis (women only); vaginitis; nongonococcal urethritis
   In the Anus or Rectum: See gonorrhea; nonspecific proctitis (men only); herpes
2. Diarrhea: See enteric STDs
3. Discharge
   From the Urethra (men only): See gonorrhea; nongonococcal urethritis; herpes
   From the Vagina (women only): See gonorrhea; herpes; warts; vaginitis; syphilis; nongonococcal urethritis

4. Fever or Aching: See gonorrhea; hepatitis; pelvic inflammatory disease (women only); syphilis
5. Growths: See warts; syphilis
6. Itching
   - In the Anus: See gonorrhea; herpes; syphilis
   - In the Vagina: See herpes; vaginitis
   - In the Genital Area: See vaginitis; crabs; scabies
   - Anywhere on the Body: See scabies; crabs
7. Rashes
   - Which Are Itchy: See vaginitis; scabies; hepatitis
   - Which Aren't Itchy: See syphilis; gonorrhea
8. Pain
   - In the Abdomen: See hepatitis; enteric STDs; pelvic inflammatory disease (women only); cystitis (women only)
   - During Intercourse: See herpes; gonorrhea; vaginitis; pelvic inflammatory disease (women only)
   - In the Testicles: See gonorrhea; nongonococcal urethritis
   - In the Joints: See hepatitis; gonorrhea
   - In the Anus: See gonorrhea; herpes; nonspecific proctitis; nongonococcal urethritis; syphilis
9. Sores: See syphilis; herpes

1: Crabs (Pubic Lice)

There is at least one famous college we know of where the clinic doctor tells anxious patients that no one has ever received a diploma there without having gone through at least one bout with crabs. Whether or not it's absolutely true, crabs *are* widespread on campuses and wherever there are sexually active people.

But there's no cause for alarm. Although they are easily spread and extremely annoying, crabs are easily cured. Regardless of how many times you contract them, they will always respond to medication. If you and the people you are intimate with all cooperate in ridding yourselves of them simultaneously and make sure that new sexual contacts are not infested, there's little reason to expect further encounters.

Mode of Transmission

Perhaps because of their appearance, many people have an inordinate fear of crabs. Examined under a magnifying glass, it's easy to see why *Pthirus pubis*—the scientific name for pubic lice—has come to be called crabs. It has a head with two big eyes and three pairs of legs with claws that are used for gripping as it scurries along.

Crabs feed on human blood and, when separated from their human host for a day or two, they will die of starvation. Because of this, they are usually spread through intimate contact with an infested person but can also be picked up from recently used sheets, clothing and, yes, toilet seats.

The female louse lays eggs on the skin that are dark brown with a hard whitish covering. The eggs, called nits, attach themselves to the hair shaft with a cement-like substance. It takes two weeks for the nits to grow into adult crabs. Both the crabs and the nits are visible to the naked eye, the crabs as moving dots and the nits as stationary whitish spots at the base of the hairs.

Symptoms

There is very little chance that you will mistake a case of crabs for anything else, since crabs look so distinctively like crabs and feel so itchy. You probably won't be looking for them, however, until the itch develops and that will occur about two to three weeks after contracting them.

The most common site is the pubic hair and groin hair, but they may also spread themselves to the hair around the anus. People who have a lot of body hair may find them crawling on the hairs of the thighs, body and underarms. In men with beards and mustaches, those are other possible sites. Finally, the eyelashes and eyebrows, especially in small children, may become infested.

The crabs are easiest to see right after feeding when the

human blood they've ingested stains them a rusty red color. The nits may be easier to spot because they are attached at the base of the pubic hair with a whitish cement-like substance.

Skin irritations may occur, caused either by excessive scratching or an especially strong sensitivity to the crabs. Some people develop bluish spots on the trunk and thighs; these aren't itchy. If crabs infest the eyelashes, the eyelids may appear swollen and crusted.

Testing for Crabs

All it takes is a magnifying glass to make a positive diagnosis for crabs. Of course, the area to look at first is the pubic region. If you have crabs there, check all the hairy spots on the body.

To estimate how long a patient has had the condition, a doctor can pluck a pubic hair with a tweezer, put it onto a slide and examine it under a microscope. Since hair grows at the rate of ¼-inch a month, the distance a nit is from the base of the hair where it is originally deposited approximates the duration of the condition. This is useful information if you want to know which of your acquaintances should be warned of possible infestation.

Treating Crabs

Crabs can generally be taken care of without a doctor's attention since there are several over-the-counter (nonprescription) medications that are as effective as prescription medications. This is definitely a case where you can save time and money by treating yourself. But you must treat yourself with one of the preparations described below; soap and water alone won't work.

There may, of course, be unusual situations where an individual is intensely reactive to crabs and develops skin inflammations that need the attention of a doctor. Or, if the condition has gone on longer than it should and itching has caused secondary bacterial infection, you will need to see a doctor.

The most common prescription medication for the treatment of crabs is lindane lotion, cream or shampoo, marketed under the brand names Kwell® or Gamene®. However, lindane isn't recommended for pregnant women or small children since it's absorbed through the skin and into the bloodstream.

Over-the-counter medications that are safe, inexpensive and effective include A200 Pyrinate,® RID® and Vonce,® just to name a few. Be sure to read the instructions in or on the package.

And don't apply any of these products around the eyes. If you or your child is infested in that area, carefully remove as many lice as possible with a tweezer. You can also buy an ophthalmic petroleum jelly product which is applied thickly twice a day for two weeks to smother remaining or hatching lice.

Applying the Medicine

If you use lotion or cream:

1. Bathe or shower and towel dry.
2. Apply a thin layer of lotion or cream to the hair around the pubis and anus. Make sure you cover it all. Then go on applying it thinly to the thighs, trunk, folds of the

underarms and groin. Remember not to use it around the eyes and don't swallow it!
3. Leave it on twenty-four hours and then wash it off thoroughly.

If you use shampoo:

1. Wet yourself thoroughly in a shower or bathtub.
2. Apply one tablespoon of shampoo to each infected area and lather for five minutes—no longer. And remember, not around the eyes or in the mouth.
3. Rinse thoroughly and towel dry.

After you've applied the medicine in one form or another, take all the clothing, towels and bed linens you've used to the laundry. They should be washed in hot water and run through a dryer on the hot cycle. Or you can have them dry cleaned. Shaving of the pubic hair is not necessary and is not recommended.

No matter what treatment you use, repeat the treatment after one week as you may still find nits attached to the hair shafts after one treatment. They have staying power. Try repeatedly running a fine-toothed comb—some medications come with combs—through the hair or picking the nits off with a tweezer. But not to the point of causing a skin inflammation—the nits have almost certainly been deactivated by the treatment. They should appear translucent because there is no larva present. That means that no new crabs will hatch from them.

The itch may persist after the lice have been destroyed because the hypersensitive reaction and the itch-scratch cycle take a while to disappear. If severe skin irritation results from excessive scratching or too frequent use of medication, see a doctor. S/he will prescribe something to ease the irritation and, if the itching has led to a secondary bacterial infection, antibiotics.

Most important, to avoid reinfestation, make certain that all your intimate contacts have also been treated. Even if they are not yet itchy, they may have crabs.

2: Cystitis

Cystitis is an inflammation of the bladder that makes you feel a desire to urinate every few minutes, but, when you try to, you feel a burning, stinging sensation and can't seem to empty your bladder completely. The condition is quite common in women.

Although cystitis is extremely uncomfortable and can easily recur, it's usually not serious and it's not even an STD. We've included it anyway because its symptoms are sometimes confused with those of other STDs such as vaginitis,* gonorrhea,* warts * and herpes.*

It can be triggered, though not transmitted, by sexual activity. Cystitis is so frequently related to a sudden increase in sexual activity that it's been nicknamed "honeymoon cystitis."

Mode of Transmission

A little physiology will explain why more women than men get cystitis (although it becomes more of a problem for men in their later years).

The bacteria which cause cystitis travel up the urethra

into the bladder, the organ that stores urine. The female urethra is shorter than the male urethra and closer to the anus.

Now, the most common cause of cystitis is *Escherichia coli (E. coli)*, bacteria which normally inhabit the large intestine and are found in fecal matter. In women, it's just a hop, skip and a jump from the anus to the urethra, and then to the bladder. In males, on the other hand, it's less likely that bacteria will be spread the distance from the anus to the urethral opening at the tip of the penis (see illustrations on pp. 3–6). And even if it is, the length of the urethra allows for the bacteria to be killed by the acidity of the urine and flushed away before it can reach the bladder.

The bladder is usually sterile and has the ability to flush out large numbers of bacteria; however, the mechanism is easily disturbed by a host of different causes and the disturbances can lead to infection. Certain groups of women are more prone to the disturbances, including older women, diabetics, pregnant women and those who are sexually active.

Symptoms

Besides the symptoms we've mentioned—the urge to urinate, the burning pain and the feeling that you can't empty your bladder (that's because it's inflamed and swollen)—you may also experience:

1. fever and chills
2. nausea and vomiting
3. diarrhea
4. blood in your urine
5. muscle tenderness and pain in the lower abdomen

Acute discomfort may indicate that the bacteria have traveled from the bladder into the kidneys, and that demands immediate medical attention.

It's possible to experience the later symptoms without ever experiencing the characteristic symptoms of cystitis. This seems particularly common in pregnant women. It's been suggested that changes in the urinary tract in late pregnancy make it especially susceptible to invasion by bacteria (if you're pregnant, see the special note at the end of this chapter).

Testing for Cystitis

Normally, with cystitis, nobody will have to tell you to go to a doctor; you'll want to get some relief. Cystitis is rarely serious, but it can be extremely uncomfortable.

The doctor will probably prescribe medication as soon as you describe your symptoms. But you should also have your urine examined to confirm the presence of bacteria. You'll be given a sterile urine collection cup.

The idea of the "clean catch" urine specimen is that any bacteria found in the specimen come only from inside the bladder. So, first wipe the area over which the urine will pass with a damp pad. Wipe from front to back to avoid contamination from the anal canal. Pass a small amount of urine into the toilet first and then fill the cup.

A drop of urine will be placed on a slide and examined for the presence of a significant amount of bacteria. Some of it may be cultured to discover the exact identity of the bacteria and its sensitivity to the medication. Don't forget to call for culture results after a day or two; you may have to change the medication originally prescribed.

Treating Cystitis

Initial attacks of cystitis respond extremely well to antibiotics. You'll probably feel better almost overnight, but you must continue to take the pills until they're finished—about two weeks. Otherwise you're inviting a recurrence and encouraging the development of strains of the bacteria that will be resistant to the medication.

For a first attack, the doctor can prescribe a number of drugs, including: sulfonamides; ampicillin (which you shouldn't take if you're allergic to penicillin drugs); and tetracycline (which shouldn't be given to pregnant women or children). If you have recurrent attacks, there are several stronger medicines which can be prescribed as alternatives. Discuss them with your doctor.

There is also a drug called phenazopyridine HCl, sold as Pyridium®, which your doctor can prescribe for you along with the antibiotic to relieve the pain and burning. It is a topical pain-killer which colors the urine reddish-orange and does the job of relieving symptoms, but it does not cure the bladder infection.

You can speed the recovery by drinking a quart of cranberry, orange, or grapefruit juice daily. Or take large doses of vitamin C. This brings the pH of your urine into the right range in order to inhibit the growth of bacteria. (But, if you're pregnant, make sure you're not ingesting too much vitamin C—more than 4 gm. a day—for the good of your baby. A fetus can become accustomed to a high vitamin C environment and develop scurvy after birth.) Include a lot of yogurt and soured milk products in your diet to counter the possibility of vaginitis,* which often results from antibiotic regimens.

There's no reason to refrain from intercourse during a bout of cystitis. But take it easy until the bladder is healed.

You may want to refrain from any positions that put a lot of pressure on the bladder, such as entry into the vagina from the rear. Using a sterile lubricant jelly may decrease irritation to the urethra.

If your symptoms haven't cleared up after a week of treatment, you should go back to your doctor. The condition may have been misdiagnosed. It may be that you have another kind of bacteria. Chlamydia has been shown to cause cystitis (see NGU *). And it may be that you don't have a bacteria infection at all. The symptoms of cystitis may result from one of the other STDs or from a physical defect in the urinary tract or its control mechanism.

If you have recurrent cystitis, it's important to get good medical attention. A doctor may prescribe low doses of an antibacterial agent over a long period of time to keep the urine sterile. If the cystitis seems to be triggered by sex, you can get antibacterial tablets that are taken before and after intercourse.

Preventing Cystitis

There are certain measures you can take to avoid the expense of doctors' visits and medications. You can consider it as a tripartite preventive program consisting of cleanliness, plenty of liquids and adequate acidity.

CLEANLINESS This means both you and your sex partners. Since cystitis is usually caused by the introduction of *E. coli* into the urethra, it stands to reason that you'd want to reduce the likelihood.

In general, of course, keep your own genital area clean. In particular, after using the toilet, wipe from front to back. Make sure your male partner washes after anal intercourse and before entering your vagina.

LIQUIDS Drink a lot of them, as a rule, and especially if you're prone to cystitis. And urinate frequently; don't ever hold urine in the bladder over long periods of time if you can help it. Urinating immediately before and after intercourse has also been suggested.

During a bout of cystitis, avoid coffee, tea, alcohol and spices. They irritate the bladder.

ACIDITY If you get cystitis regularly, it may mean that the relative acidity of your urine is too low to kill bacteria. You can bring the acidity up by taking a lot of vitamin C or drinking cranberry or other citrus juices daily. Buy some phenaphithazine paper in a drugstore to check the pH of your urine. It costs about $5.00 a roll. It will come with instructions. The lower the pH, the higher the acidity. If you find that the pH is above 5.0, bring it down with vitamin C and juices.

Cystitis and Pregnancy

If you are pregnant, get your urine tested for bacteria even if you have none of the symptoms of cystitis. Undetected bacteria in the urine during pregnancy has been related to premature births.

Treatment during pregnancy is similar to what is generally recommended. Make sure your doctor knows you are pregnant so that s/he can prescribe the safest medication. You should ask for follow-up cultures during and after pregnancy.

3: Enteric STDs (Shigellosis, Amebiasis, Giardiasis)

UP UNTIL RECENTLY it was supposed that about the only way to get an intestinal parasite was to visit a foreign country and swallow food or water contaminated with fecal material containing the organisms.

Now, however, enteric (or intestinal) diseases are being transmitted in America among people who haven't been traveling. By far the three most common ones are shigellosis, amebiasis and giardiasis. The male homosexual community, particularly in large urban centers like New York and San Francisco, appears to be at highest risk, although there's no reason at all to dismiss the possibility of enteric STDs on the grounds that you're female or heterosexual. Anybody's eligible depending on sexual practices (we'll discuss that in more detail in the section on transmission).

This is all so new that the medical establishment has not quite caught up with the phenomenon yet. Tropical disease clinics, which have traditionally treated these diseases, are being heavily strained. Most private physicians, on the other hand, don't have experience in diagnosing and treating enteric pathogens. The symptoms of these diseases can be easily confused with other sorts of intestinal problems.

It's important that if, after reading the following description, you think you might have one of the enteric STDs, you visit a doctor who is knowledgeable and to whom you can talk openly about your sexual practices.

Mode of Transmission

Any form of sexual activity that results in the swallowing of even the tiniest amount of contaminated fecal material could lead to an enteric STD. This of course includes oral-anal contact, which is often called "rimming." But it can include a lot of other activities, since the organisms that cause the diseases can survive as long as a week on moist surfaces outside the body. They can be carried on fingers, towels, sheets, food, etc. Unfortunately, there is often no way of knowing whether a person is carrying an enteric pathogen, since most of the carriers are asymptomatic.

Shigellosis is caused by bacteria, while both amebiasis and giardiasis are caused by protozoa. The protozoa that causes amebiasis is called *Entamoeba histolytica* (sometimes amebiasis is called amebic dysentery). Giardiasis is caused by *Giardia lamblia.*

Amebiasis and giardiasis are spread when the protozoa is in a particular form—the cyst form. The cysts are passed through the stools of the infected person. If swallowed by another person, they pass through the stomach and into the small intestines where the protective walls that enclose the cysts disintegrate and release a number of trophozoites, between four and eight each. The trophozoites are the active, feeding form of the organism, and it is they who produce the symptoms of the diseases. But they can't transmit the disease from one individual to another; that is done by the cysts.

Symptoms

For amebiasis, giardiasis and shigellosis, the symptoms are very similar. They can be so mild as to escape attention or severe enough to send a person to the hospital, but they tend to fall under the general category of gastro-intestinal distress. Symptoms can include:

1. Diarrhea or increased frequency of bowel movements. For the two protozoal infections, this can alternate with normal bowel movements or even constipation.
2. Abdominal cramps and gas.
3. Nausea and vomiting.
4. Fever and chills with shigellosis.
5. Straining of the stools; a sense of having to defecate all the time.
6. The stools may be liquid and greenish, watery and foul-smelling and may contain mucus and blood.
7. Dehydration may result if the diarrhea is severe.
8. Any persistent change from your normal bowel movements.

Shigellosis tends to feel more brutal and explosive than the two protozoal infections, but they too can have an extremely debilitating effect, especially on people in a generally weakened condition.

Testing for Enteric STDs

It's almost impossible to distinguish between an enteric STD and various forms of other bowel diseases on the basis of symptoms alone. But it's extremely important to make the correct diagnosis since medication, which is often administered for some forms of colitis (i.e., cortisone), can make a protozoal infection even worse.

The average doctor will probably not think to test you for enteric pathogens unless s/he knows something about sexual modes of transmission and is also aware that your sexual practices put you at risk for contacting them. You should feel comfortable enough with the doctor to discuss your individual situation and your suspicions. You're more likely to find a knowledgeable and sympathetic doctor in a large urban area where the incidence of this sort of STD is higher or in the tropical disease or parasitology department of a large hospital, which also has the laboratory facilities for proper testing.

Proper testing for amebiasis and giardiasis means careful examination of a series of stool specimens immediately after they've been passed. The lab technician will be looking for ova and parasites. To test for shigellosis you will need a bacterial stool culture.

Make sure your doctor sends you to a laboratory that specializes in stool testing. It is critical to have a good lab since it's relatively difficult with the enteric pathogens to make a correct diagnosis. For best results, stools should be examined within an hour of passage. It is possible to preserve a cold stool sample and examine it later, but that method is considered less sensitive and may give false negative results.

Before visiting the lab, don't take enemas, antibiotics, anti-diarrhea medications, or antacid preparations, since these substances interfere with the isolation and identification of the pathogens. Be prepared to spend some money: each lab visit should cost about $30 and, if you have the disease, you will have to repeat the test at least once.

If you know you are at risk for the enteric STDs—because, for example, other people you know have them—

don't jump into expensive gastro-intestinal tests without having had a freshly purged stool test. They could wind up costing thousands of dollars.

Treating Enteric STDs

If you have one of the three diseases described in this chapter, you're probably feeling weak and disgusted and a little depressed. Well, it may feel worse before it feels better, but summon up your strength and pull yourself together. It will be important to take all your medicine and make a strong effort to protect yourself from reinfection—because reinfection can occur easily if you're not careful, and medication becomes less effective in recurrences.

Shigellosis, since it's caused by bacteria, is treated with antibiotics. There are a number of choices depending on the strain of the shigella bacteria. Ampicillin is the preferred medication, but other possibilities include tetracycline and trimethoprim-sulfamethoxazole.

For giardiasis, there are two possibilities. The treatment of choice is quinacrine (Atabrine®). Metronidazole (Flagyl®) is also effective against giardiasis, but it has one major drawback. It has been shown to cause cancer and tumors in animals when administered in large doses. While there is no proof that it affects humans that way, there doesn't seem to be reason to risk it so long as there are other effective medications.

Amebiasis, on the other hand, is usually treated with metronidazole; it's the drug which seems most effective and least harmful. It's given in a relatively high dose for ten days together with another drug, diiodohydroxyquin. Metronidazole can cause depression and nausea, so be prepared and determined. It's very important to take all the medication even though you may not be feeling like it. And don't drink alcoholic beverages during treatment.

If you're absolutely opposed to metronidazole, ask your doctor about Humatin.® It's an expensive alternative at about $70 per treatment.

You're likely to need lots of rest; lengthy bouts of diarrhea can be very exhausting. You also will want to make sure you replace the fluid and minerals you lose. Drink a lot of juices and broths so you won't become seriously dehydrated.

You'll have an appointment for a follow-up stool test. Until you're sure that the tests are negative, don't participate in any sexual activity that might spread the disease. And be very careful with your personal hygiene. Wash your hands thoroughly with soap and water after going to the toilet and scrub your nails with a nail brush.

Very, very important is the need to make sure that any recent sexual partners undergo the laboratory test. The fact that they're not feeling sick is absolutely no indication that they're not carrying the disease. And as long as they are carrying it, they are spreading it, perhaps back in your direction.

4: Gonorrhea

YOU MAY KNOW IT as The Clap, A Dose, A Strain, G.C. But you probably don't know that it's almost as popular as the common cold. If you've got it, you're in plenty of company. It's epidemic in the United States, striking about once every twelve seconds, or at the rate of 2.7 million annually.

So chances are pretty good that you have been or will be in contact with someone, some time, who has gonorrhea, even though they show absolutely no signs of it. And then, the possibility that you'll pick it up from them is quite good in men, even better in women, since the cervix is extremely conducive to the growth of *Neisseria gonorrhoeae*, the bacteria which causes the disease.

A Kcy to the Subchapters

We've divided this chapter into five sections based on the locations of the infection:

1. In the cervix (women only): Cervical Gonorrhea, see p. 36

2. In the urethra (men only): Urethral Gonorrhea, see p. 38
3. In the anus: Anal Gonorrhea, see p. 40
4. In the throat: Pharyngeal Gonorrhea, see p. 41
5. In the eyes: Gonococcal Conjunctivitis, see p. 42

A General Introduction

No matter where in the body gonorrhea occurs, testing and treating are essentially the same (where there are differences, we'll indicate them in the subchapters). And if you have gonorrhea in one place, you may have it in other places as well. For instance, heterosexual males are more likely to contract urethral gonorrhea. But then they may also have pharyngeal gonorrhea, and this has led researchers to assume that it's possible to contract it through oral contact with an infected area.

Gay males have a higher incidence of both anal and pharyngeal gonorrhea, but they also have a high rate of urethral gonorrhea. Cervical gonorrhea, with all its special problems, is reserved for women, but they are certainly not exempted from pharyngeal or anal gonorrhea.

Gonorrhea is tricky. Its primary symptoms are usually much clearer in men than they are in women. But often, for both sexes, it appears to be something else, or doesn't appear at all—until later, when complications set in. Complications most typically involve the reproductive organs and may result in sterility. In a small percentage of cases the bacteria spreads into the bloodstream and from there may localize in the joints, causing arthritis. It may also spread to the heart or the liver, a situation which may be fatal. All of this, of course, can be avoided by early diagnosis and treatment.

So, even if there are no signs at all and none of your

sexual partners have mentioned any problems to you, it's smart to have yourself tested regularly for gonorrhea. The test is offered free or for a small fee at public clinics. Or you can get it from your doctor for an additional $5 to $10.

And if you know you've been intimate with someone who has gonorrhea, go to a doctor or clinic as soon as possible. The incubation period is quite short, usually around three to five days. If you have it treated then, you can prevent the disease altogether. Preventive treatment is the same as regular treatment, only earlier.

Testing for Gonorrhea

The most common test for gonorrhea is called the Gram stain. It's most useful in detecting urethral gonorrhea in men with symptoms. A sample of discharge is examined for gonococcal bacteria. Under a microscope the gonococci look like little beans in pairs, each pair enclosed in a pus cell. If the discharge is positive for gonococci, medication will start immediately. This is the time to tell your sex partners about the problem so they may have themselves treated.

If the Gram stain test is negative, however, it's still quite possible that you have gonorrhea and that the gonococci haven't yet emerged from the incubatory stage. Or they may somehow have managed to elude that particular specimen, as is frequently the case with cervical, anal and pharyngeal gonorrhea. A culture test should always be done when a Gram stain test comes out negative. And men who have a discharge should always begin medication in any case (see nongonococcal urethritis *).

The Gram stain is a simple test; clinics and doctors who see many STD patients do it for all patients as a rule. But most doctors don't have the facilities to process the culture test. The test consists of placing a sample from the infected site onto a little plate that contains the "medium" and watching it for growth of gonococci. The doctor can do the initial work, but then it is sent to a laboratory. So it will take a few days to get the final results, but it is worth waiting for because then you will know for sure. Until you have gotten word on the test, use a condom or don't have sex.

If the culture is negative, gonorrhea is ruled out. If it is positive, you will be treated for gonorrhea. Three to seven days after completion of treatment, another culture, called the "test of cure," will be performed to make sure the medication has done the job.

Once in a great while, the medication doesn't cure the infection and the patient has to be treated again. But most often when the treatment doesn't work, reinfection from a sex partner who's got gonorrhea has occurred. Then it's return to go!

Treating Gonorrhea

First things first: From the moment you suspect you have gonorrhea until the moment you receive a negative result for your "test of cure," you should take special care to protect others who come in contact with you. Avoid sex before treatment. After treatment and before you receive your "test of cure" result, use condoms during vaginal and anal intercourse and refrain from penile-oral intercourse. Make sure that your sexual partners have themselves tested and take your children, if you have any, for an examination. This is the first and most important line of defense (see section on gonorrhea and children).

Second, there's the medication. Procaine penicillin is extremely effective in most cases. It's injected in one large dose into each of the buttocks. At the same time, you will receive an oral drug, probenecid, which lengthens the time the penicillin stays in the bloodstream.

Ampicillin and amoxicillin are oral penicillin drugs that can be taken in a single dose and are increasingly used instead of penicillin injections. They are just as effective, except in cases of gonorrhea of the throat, where injected penicillin is most effective.

If you are allergic to penicillin, you'll receive either spectinomycin, which is injected, or tetracycline. Tetracycline is taken orally, and should be taken on an empty stomach an hour before or two hours after meals. Also, avoid dairy products because they interfere with its absorption into the body.

If you are pregnant *and* allergic to penicillin, you shouldn't use tetracycline; it may cause liver problems as well as staining your baby's teeth. One alternative, erythromycin, doesn't have such side-effects. Neither does spectinomycin, although it hasn't yet been declared completely safe for pregnant women.

PPNG, or penicillinase-producing *N. gonorrhoeae,* is a strain of gonorrhea which seems to have developed in Southeast Asia and to have been brought into this country during and after the Vietnam War. It caused a great deal of alarm at first because it is resistant to the usual treatment with penicillin. But it's been discovered that PPNG responds to other medications such as spectinomycin and cefoxitin. And it's not very widespread here. Thus, it's no more, or less, alarming than the other strains of gonorrhea.

Gonorrhea and Children

Adults can pass gonorrhea on to very young children unintentionally while bathing together or through towels freshly contaminated with gonococcal discharge. Little girls especially are susceptible to vaginal gonorrhea. They will develop a heavy discharge and inflammation of the area.

If a young child develops gonorrhea, it's also possible that s/he has been sexually abused. In any case, if you are a parent with young children and find that you or a sex partner have gonorrhea, it's a good idea to have your children checked for it.

All pregnant women should receive routine gonorrhea cultures, both at the initial obstetrical visit and in the last weeks of pregnancy. Ask for it. Gonorrhea in pregnancy is dangerous, to both mother and infant, especially if the mother has gonorrhea at the time of childbirth. Both mothers and infants with gonorrhea appear to have a higher incidence of illness and death.

The most common cause of blindness in babies used to be cervical gonorrhea in the pregnant mother. As the baby passes out of the body, it contracts the disease in its eyes. But now, the routine use in most hospitals of either ointment or drops in the baby's eyes has made this less likely.

Cervical Gonorrhea

Mode of Transmission

The cervix is the passageway high up in the vaginal canal which marks the entrance to the uterus (see illustration on pp. 5–6). It can easily be reached with a finger (it protrudes a bit from the back wall of the vagina) or seen with a speculum. If you've had intercourse with a man who may have urethral gonorrhea, please read the following carefully.

Symptoms

It's been estimated that about 80 percent of women with cervical gonorrhea don't know it. If there is a discharge, most women don't notice it. If they do, they may think it's one of a number of other diseases, such as vaginitis,* herpes,* warts * or syphilis.* Usually the discharge is thick and yellowish, but it may also be thin. If the gonococci have also invaded the urethra, there may be burning during urination, but this is not as common in women as it is in men. Burning on urination may also indicate cystitis.*

The speculum is extremely useful in detecting changes in the cervix (see Appendix A). If you have gonorrhea, you may, using the speculum, see a thick discharge, redness in the area, and the cervix itself may appear covered with small bumps which doctors call granular erosions.

Testing and Treatment

If you have any suspicions whatever of having gonorrhea, have a cervical culture done. It is the only way to detect the infection in women. A Gram stain smear is not very sensitive in detecting cervical gonorrhea. Some gynecologists suggest to their sexually active patients that they be tested every three or four months routinely. This is because there are serious complications.

If cervical gonorrhea is allowed to spread to the reproductive organs, a woman will develop pelvic inflammatory disease * (PID). About half of all women who get PID, even once, find their fertility impaired. And besides that, it hurts.

As part of your routine gynecological examination, you should be cultured for gonorrhea. And checked for PID. The procedure for that, which is quite simple, is a bimanual pelvic examination. It's explained in detail in the chapter on PID.

During the few days it takes to get the culture results, avoid vaginal intercourse so as not to spread the infection. And if the test comes back positive, your sex partners should be examined whether or not they show signs of gonorrhea.

It's been found that barrier forms of contraception, such as a diaphragm or foam, and especially the condom, are very effective in lessening the chances of infection. On the other hand, low-estrogen birth control pills change the chemical balance of the vaginal wall from acidic to basic, encouraging the growth of gonococci.

Urethral Gonorrhea

Mode of Transmission

The urethra in the male is the narrow passageway in the penis through which sperm and urine travel (see illustrations on p. 3–4). It's the most common site of gonococcal infection in men. If your urethra has made contact with a cervix, an anus or possibly even a throat that's infected, you may develop urethral gonorrhea.

Symptoms

You should know within a few days, because there will be an intense burning during urination (during the Middle Ages, the disease was well known simply as "the burning"). There's also a discharge, which can be thin and clear or thick and creamy and can vary in color from yellowish to greenish.

These symptoms are similar to those for nongonococcal urethritis * (NGU), but they are usually worse for gonorrhea. The culture test is the only sure way to differentiate between the two. Men who've contracted trichomoniasis (see chapter on vaginitis *), herpes * or urethral warts * may also have a discharge, but in those cases it's more likely to itch than to burn.

It's also possible to be asymptomatic, not to notice any symptoms. Or the symptoms may be "masked" if you are taking antibiotics for another condition. But the antibiotics may not be strong enough to cure the gonorrhea, so it's important to tell your doctor if you are taking antibiotics when you are tested.

In any case, symptoms tend to go away within a couple of months. But the disease if untreated will be there nonetheless, with the possibility of its spreading into the bloodstream. The most common complications of untreated urethral gonorrhea appear in the reproductive organs. There may be swelling in the testicles, swelling and pain in the penis, abscesses and scarring in the urethra.

The greatest hazard is urethral scarring. Scarring narrows the urethral passage so that, eventually, if someone has repeated bouts with gonorrhea, he will find urination difficult and painful. Urethral scarring also leads to sterility. The condition can sometimes be corrected surgically.

Testing and Treatment

Testing and treatment are explained in the introduction to this chapter. If you still have a discharge after treatment, you may have a form of NGU * called postgonococcal urethritis (PGU). Make sure that all your sexual partners are tested too.

Anal Gonorrhea

Mode of Transmission

Gonococci enter the anus in two ways: during penile-anal intercourse and through auto-inoculation. Anyone who takes a receptive role in penile-anal intercourse may contract it from a man with urethral gonorrhea. In many women who have cervical gonorrhea it spreads via discharge from the vagina (auto-inoculation). So it's important to be tested for anal gonorrhea at the same time you're tested for cervical gonorrhea.

Symptoms

Most people don't have any symptoms for anal gonorrhea. When there are symptoms, there may be a slight rectal burn, mucus in the stools or an itch which goes away eventually although the gonococci don't and can still be spread to others.

In a small number of people the symptoms will be more dramatic: a profuse anal discharge, a sensation of anal fullness, severe pain on defecation or pus and blood in the stools. However, all of these symptoms are common to other problems such as anal abscesses, nonspecific proctitis,* enteric infections,* anal herpes * and syphilis.* The only way to be sure that it is or is not anal gonorrhea is to be tested.

Testing and Treatment

The person doing the examination should use an anoscope. An anoscope is a small plastic instrument which, when inserted into the anus, allows for visual examination and the taking of specimens. In some cases the examiner will simply use a cotton-tipped swab. Both anoscope and swab are relatively painless unless the symptoms are severe.

You must have a culture done for anal gonorrhea, since the Gram stain test is not very sensitive in this case. Even if the Gram stain is negative, wait for the results of your culture to be sure.

Refer to the introduction to this chapter for a description of treatment.

Pharyngeal Gonorrhea

Mode of Transmission

There are a lot of uncertainties about how gonococci are transmitted to the throat and whether they can then be transmitted from the throat to other areas. In terms of hard statistics, pharyngeal gonorrhea occurs most frequently in people who have penile-oral sex (fellatio; "sucking"), but it has been seen occasionally in people who don't.

It appears unlikely that it's spread during oral-vaginal sex (cunnilingus; "eating") or from an infected anus during oral-rectal sex (anilingus; "rimming"). Neither is it thought to be spread from throat to throat during deep-kissing. But too little research has been done to reach definite conclusions.

Symptoms

Most people with gonorrhea of the throat aren't even aware they have it. Some people notice a mild sore throat, and very few experience severe inflammation.

Testing and Treatment

The Gram stain is of no value for pharyngeal gonorrhea; be sure to have a specimen from your throat cultured when you are tested for gonorrhea, especially if you engage in fellatio, cunnilingus or anilingus.

Oral forms of penicillin are ineffective with pharyngeal gonorrhea; it must be injected. If you're allergic to penicillin, tetracycline is generally thought to be effective.

Gonococcal Conjunctivitis (or Gonococcal Ophthalmia)

Mode of Transmission

The conjunctiva is the mucous membrane that lines the inner surface of the eyelid and the exposed surface of the eyeball. It's particularly susceptible to gonococcal infection if it comes in contact with discharge from an infected area.

Adults contract gonococcal conjunctivitis by touching their eyes with anything that is carrying the discharge. For example, towels, sheets, or fingers with fresh discharge can transfer the infection.

As we've mentioned earlier, gonococci used to be the chief cause of infants contracting ophthalmia neonatorum, which can result in blindness. Now, infants' eyes are treated routinely in most places at birth with silver nitrate drops or penicillin. Another important preventive measure is testing all pregnant women for gonorrhea.

Many other organisms can cause conjunctivitis, but if there is the least bit of suspicion of gonorrhea, the Gram stain and culture should be done immediately, since serious complications develop quickly.

Symptoms

Within two to four days of infection the eyes start swelling and reddening. There is a pus discharge which gets thicker as the infection develops. If it isn't treated immediately, the cornea can become severely damaged and the damage can result in blindness.

Testing and Treatment

Testing for gonococcal conjunctivitis includes the routine tests but, whatever the results, if gonorrhea is suspected medication begins immediately. Adults receive injections for five days running or as long as it takes to clear up the infection. During this time, drops or ointment are also applied to the eyes. Both parts of the treatment must be performed; neither one is sufficient by itself.

Children receive their medication intravenously rather than by injection, so it's usually necessary for them to be hospitalized for a short time.

5: Hepatitis

HEPATITIS SIMPLY MEANS an inflammation of the liver. A liver can become inflamed in many different ways, but more and more often hepatitis is being caused by viruses that are transmitted sexually.

Jaundice—a condition in which the skin and whites of the eyes acquire a yellowish tint—is a hot tip that a person may have hepatitis. Jaundice occurs when the liver is unable to filter bile pigment properly.

However, over 50 percent of people with hepatitis contract mild cases, so mild that jaundice doesn't occur. Mild hepatitis often resembles a cold or the flu.

It's also possible to contract the virus, but be totally without symptoms (asymptomatic). If you carry the virus, whether or not you show symptoms, you may be spreading it to others. Sexually active individuals should consider periodic tests for hepatitis to be sure they aren't spreading the virus unknowingly.

Mode of Transmission

There are several different viruses responsible for the transmission of hepatitis. These forms of hepatitis produce similar symptoms but each is spread in a slightly different way:

HEPATITIS A Hepatitis A used to be called infectious hepatitis. It's caused by a virus that's found in the feces of infected individuals. Obviously, any kind of sexual activity that involves swallowing even tiny quantities of feces can spread the disease. Those at high risk for sexually acquired hepatitis A are people who participate in anal-oral sex (commonly called "rimming") or rectal intercourse followed by oral sex.

It's also possible to contract hepatitis A nonsexually, from food or water containing contaminated fecal material. Raw clams or oysters are a particularly common source of the infection.

The incubation period for the disease is about one month. It can be prevented in most people *if they receive an injection of immune serum globulin within two weeks following exposure.* Immune serum globulin (ISG or gamma globulin) is made from the blood serum of individuals who've had hepatitis A before and have therefore developed antibodies to the disease. Sometimes ISG doesn't completely prevent the disease, but even then it will lessen the severity. So, if you think you've been exposed to hepatitis A, go get your injection.

HEPATITIS B Hepatitis B used to be called serum hepatitis. It's caused by a virus present in the blood and all the bodily fluids—saliva, semen, sweat, urine, menstrual blood and vaginal secretions—of infected individuals. This means, of course, that any kind of intimate contact, including kissing, can spread the disease. Shared razors, toothbrushes, towels and other intimate articles can also spread the virus.

While hepatitis B can be contracted by both men and women, some researchers think that there is a sex-linked factor which makes men somewhat more susceptible. Sexually active gay men seem to be at particularly high risk.

Type B hepatitis can be carried and spread by a person who has no symptoms at all. In fact, most hepatitis B carriers appear totally healthy. A person who has had the symptoms of hepatitis can be carrying and spreading the virus long after the symptoms have disappeared.

The incubation period for hepatitis B is one to six months, two months on the average. There is a special form of immune serum globulin for hepatitis B (hepatitis B ISG), which can prevent or lessen the severity of the disease. But it's quite expensive, about $150 per treatment.

Prior infection with hepatitis A doesn't prevent infection with hepatitis B, and vice versa. But an attack of either one *will* provide immunity to that same type in the future.

HEPATITIS NON A NON B Hepatitis Non A Non B is caused by viruses which, as the name suggests, are neither A nor B. What exactly they are is not yet clear. Up until recently it wasn't regarded as sexually transmissible. It's still more commonly associated with blood transfusions, but lately it's been noticed increasingly among sexually active young adults who've never had a blood transfusion.

So far, there's little to say about prevention of hepatitis non A non B. It's not yet known whether immune serum globulin is effective.

Symptoms

The symptoms of hepatitis in those who develop jaundice can be identified in three stages: pre-jaundice; jaundice;

recovery. Generally, hepatitis A starts suddenly while hepatitis B tends to descend gradually.

The Pre-jaundice Stage

1. Flu-like symptoms, including: a cough; sore throat; runny nose.
2. Usually a severe loss of appetite; fatigue; a feeling of listlessness; and weakness.
3. Sometimes nausea; joint and muscle aches and a mild fever.
4. Sometimes with type B, hives and pains in the joints.

The Jaundice Stage

1. The urine darkens to brownish.
2. The stools become light and clay-colored.
3. The skin and the whites of the eyes turn yellowish.
4. There is soreness in the abdomen, on the upper right hand side.
5. General itchiness.
6. Severe weakness and loss of stamina.

The Recovery Stage

The jaundice may last from two to eight weeks. Recovery from hepatitis A tends to be quicker than recovery from hepatitis B. The stools turn darker, the yellowish tint in the skin and eyes fades, the urine lightens and other flu-like or gastro-intestinal symptoms disappear.

After the jaundice clears up, it may take a while to feel normal again. Weight losses of five to ten pounds during hepatitis are quite common. It's usual during the recovery stage to continue feeling tired. It may take three to four months before the liver is functioning normally, and it may take six months to a year before one feels completely healthy again.

Testing for Hepatitis

If you suspect that you have any of the forms of hepatitis, or have been exposed to them recently, see a doctor. After doing the proper urine and blood tests, the doctor will be able to tell you:

1. what kind of hepatitis you have;
2. the extent of liver dysfunction;
3. how long you should expect to be infectious.

Don't be shy about asking questions!

There is a widely available test for the hepatitis B surface antigen (HB_sAg). If you test positively for it and your liver function tests show that your liver is dysfunctioning, you will be treated for an active case of hepatitis B.

If you test positive for HB_sAg repeatedly over an extended length of time, say six months after the symptoms have disappeared, you are considered a hepatitis B carrier, capable of spreading the disease. This happens in a few but not many cases.

While there is no specific test for the hepatitis A virus, there is a blood test that measures an immunological response that can be triggered by the body in reaction to the hepatitis A virus. If the hepatitis B test is negative, but this test is positive, your doctor may conclude that you have hepatitis A.

If hepatitis A and hepatitis B are ruled out, although tests show that the liver is not functioning correctly, and you have the symptoms of the disease, then another form of hepatitis is indicated.

Now, there are several types of blood tests that monitor liver function. Tests for SGOT, SGPT, alkaline phosphatase, LDH and the total bilirubin levels measure the amounts of liver enzymes and bilirubin (bile pigment) in the blood. An increase in these indicate that the liver is diseased and unable to purify the blood properly. The higher the level, the bigger the problem. If you are recuperating from hepatitis, you can ask your doctor for the test results and watch the scores decline.

Unfortunately, hepatitis is a relatively expensive proposition because the laboratory tests have to be repeated to make sure your liver is healing properly. Be prepared to spend a couple of hundred dollars and maybe more.

Treating Hepatitis

Vaccines for hepatitis are currently being tested, but for now the only treatment is simple and old-fashioned: plenty of rest and good, healthy food. The point is to treat your body as well as possible and give it the strength to fight the invading virus.

You may be quite tired during your bout. It's not necessary to stay in bed constantly, but allow yourself all the rest you need, particularly after meals. Your physical activity will probably need to be curtailed somewhat, depending of course on how active a person you normally are. Forget about jogging and stay away from discos for awhile. It's important not to exhaust yourself.

You *must* eat your meals. Your appetite will probably be

very small but it's absolutely essential to get the nutrients your body needs. Keep eating, many small meals if necessary, but keep eating. Your diet should be balanced and as high in calories as you can make it.

Don't take *any* kind of medication until you've cleared it with your doctor. Even aspirin—it may cause gastro-intestinal bleeding. Drinking alcohol is also out—alcoholic beverages strain the liver even in the best of times. Wait until your doctor says that your liver is well enough to start handling alcohol again. That might take six months or longer.

Some doctors prescribe steroids. They do relieve some of the symptoms, but they are potent and potentially dangerous. And they don't cure hepatitis.

Don't be discouraged. It can feel like an awfully long haul with no miracle drug for instant health. But the human body is a pretty miraculous organism and given the rest and nutrition it needs, will probably do the job of healing within weeks or months. A very small percentage of people experience a mild relapse within a half year, and an even smaller percentage develop chronic hepatitis. But these are very few.

Pregnancy and Hepatitis

Hepatitis doesn't necessarily have to affect pregnancy and child-bearing adversely. Of course, it does mean that rest and good nutrition are doubly important, both to cure the disease and to support the growth of the fetus.

There are some serious risks however. Hepatitis early in pregnancy increases the possibility of spontaneous abortion. Later in pregnancy it increases the possibility of premature labor. Mothers with active cases of hepatitis B, or who are hepatitis B carriers, often deliver infants who are hepatitis B carriers.

Immune serum globulin is safe for pregnant women and infants. ISG should be given to a pregnant woman as soon as possible after exposure to hepatitis. Infants born to mothers with positive tests for hepatitis B should be given hepatitis B ISG.

6: Herpes

THE HERPES SIMPLEX VIRUS, which comes in two strains—HSV I and HSV II—has been causing a great deal of concern lately. It's spreading rather quickly with no sure-fire cure in sight.

Herpes in the genital area is getting the most attention because it's linked with cervical cancer in women. Studies indicate that women with genital herpes have a five times greater risk of developing cervical cancer.

While this is unquestionably alarming information for any woman who has herpes—or, for that matter, any woman at all who is having sex with more than one partner—it's important to remember that *cervical cancer can be cured if detected early. Women with herpes should get a Pap test every six months.* (There are several organizations which offer free testing. Consult your local American Cancer Society office.)

In any case, herpes is often a painful, stress-provoking and tiresome bother for men and women alike. Once a person is infected with either form of the virus, there are periodic recurrences of the herpes sores for life. A brighter point is that the recurrences are less severe than the first infection; they heal faster and diminish in frequency with time.

Mode of Transmission

Both strains of the herpes virus can travel anywhere in the body but they seem to have different geographical preferences. HSV I is generally found above the waist, whereas HSV II tends to settle in the genital area. But this is not a hard and fast rule. Oral-genital and oral-anal sex as well as transmission via the fingers can spread herpes from its natural habitat to another.

The infection is initially contracted when the virus penetrates one of the thin membranes of the genitalia, the anus or the mouth. There must be direct contact with the herpes sores or the secretions of an infected person.

The herpes infection is much more active and transmissible during those times when somebody with herpes has the sores. The fluid secreted from an open herpetic sore is by far the most virulent medium of transmission. But a person whose herpes is in a latent stage may still transmit the virus through the saliva, semen or vaginal secretions.

HSV I is the cause of the common cold sores usually found on the gums, tongue and lips. It's most often caught before an individual is five years old. People with HSV I who contract HSV II later on in life, tend to get less severe attacks of herpes II.

Symptoms

Both herpes I and herpes II produce painful, fluid-filled blisters which break to form crusty sores. In the first attack, called the primary attack, the sores occur about one week (from two to twenty days) after exposure to the virus. They last about two to three weeks and heal completely, leaving no scars.

There is usually at least one recurrence within six months of the primary attack, but the recurrences are less frequent and milder as time goes on. The repeats occur in the same spot as the primary attack. Often, people with genital herpes can feel a burning, tingling or painful sensation in the area before a recurrence.

While the primary attack is usually fairly severe, it *is* possible to be completely unaware of it. If the sores are internal, there may be no pain at all. In women with HSV II, the sores are frequently on the cervix, which is insensitive to pain.

The following is a description of a primary attack of genital herpes by site of infection (refer to illustrations on pp. 3–6):

- *On the head or shaft of the penis or in the urethra.* Uncircumcised men may get sores around the foreskin. If the infection is in the urethra, there may be burning on urination, a urethral discharge or an inflammation of the prostate gland.
- *On the cervix or anywhere in a woman's genital area,* including the labia, vagina, urethra or perineum.
- *Pelvic and systemic.* In a severe primary attack, the entire pelvic region may ache. This is not unusual for women. Some people may have a fever, headache and swollen glands.
- *In the anus* (otherwise known as herpetic proctitis). There may be severe pain, burning and itching. If the sores spread, there may be swollen glands in the genital region. Other possible symptoms include: constipation and general urinary difficulty; abdominal pain; pain in

the buttocks and upper thighs; general feeling of ill health; impotence.

- *The eyes.*
  This usually happens when somebody who has herpes sores touches his/her own eyes, but it may also be transmitted from one person to another. It can have some serious effects—an inflammation of the cornea, called herpetic keratitis or herpetic conjunctivitis, which may lead to blindness. Fortunately, both these conditions can be successfully treated if diagnosed soon enough.

Testing for Herpes

An attack of herpes can usually be identified on sight. Tests are necessary if the lesions are on the cervix, in the urethra or in the vagina, or if the infection is subclinical—there aren't any lesions but the herpes virus is present in the system. Also to make sure that the condition is definitely herpes and not another STD, such as syphilis *—the sores can resemble herpes—and gonorrhea.*

There are several laboratory tests that isolate the herpes virus. For the Tzanck test, a sample of fluid collected from a sore is smeared on a slide and examined for the virus.

The Pap smear, usually performed to screen for the presence of cervical cancer, is also used routinely in detecting cervical herpes. This is often the only way a woman with asymptomatic cervical herpes can find out she has it. It's information any woman who is planning to have children should have.

Then there are blood tests which identify antibodies that the body manufactures to fight the herpes virus. They're of limited value, however, because lots of people who've been exposed to herpes develop antibodies but don't become herpes virus carriers.

Treating Herpes

At this point in time, there is no safe, effective treatment for use against genital herpes that has been approved by the Food and Drug Administration. There are a number of substances now being investigated and preliminary trials show some good results. But there is nothing definite as yet to say, however much we'd like to.

A word about a process which has been used in the past—it's called photodynamic inactivation. Some experts now feel that the process itself may cause cells to become malignant. Its use is no longer recommended. If you've ever had the therapy, check the area periodically for changes in the skin, growths, or sores, and see a doctor if anything develops.

Ocular herpes is the only form of herpes which can be treated successfully with medication if detected at an early stage. Three alternative prescription medicines for topical application are 5-iododeoxyuridine, adenine arabinoside or trifluorothymidine.

IN THE MEANTIME, there are a number of things you can do for yourself which won't cure the herpes, but might make your situation less uncomfortable. You'll have to tailor the advice to your own needs, since what suits some won't satisfy others.

1. It's generally a good idea to keep the infected area clean and dry. This may help to contain the sores in one place, speed the healing process and discourage secondary bacterial infection. Some drying agents you can try are alcohol, ketone and Burrow's compress.
2. Sitting in a hot sitz bath may bring relief, especially with a severe primary attack.

3. Avoid tight clothing which rubs against the sores, and nylon underwear or pantyhose which trap moisture.
4. If your sores are located in an area where they are being irritated by urine, try applying a small amount of petroleum jelly to cover them. But be sure to remove it after you've urinated.
3. If the sores are very painful, a topical anesthetic like Xylocaine ointment may make you more comfortable.

Help

The American Social Health Association offers a service for people infected with herpes. It's called HELP. Because herpes often causes a great deal of anxiety in those who contract it, and because anxiety is precisely what one wants to avoid since it may aggravate the herpes, HELP is dedicated to reducing the psychological component through self-help and support groups. HELP provides its members with a quarterly newsletter which contains detailed medical information and current research on herpes. If you'd like to know more about the organization write to: HELP/ Box 100/ Palo Alto, Calif. 94302.

Protecting Yourself and Others

Herpes recurrences can be triggered in many different ways. The particular situations vary from person to person, but include moisture, sunburn, exposure to ultraviolet light, fatigue, traumatic events, illness, certain drugs, menstruation and stress. You can try to analyze the cases of herpes you have had to see what's triggered them and then, if possible, avoid repeating the situation.

In general, avoiding extreme stress is a good idea. There

are a great many good books written these days on techniques for combatting stress, finding a proper diet and strengthening the body's defense mechanisms. If you have herpes, you may be able to decrease the frequency and intensity of the attacks through these means.

To protect others, you may want to consider using a barrier contraceptive during sex. There are many different condoms from which you can choose (see Appendix C). During the times when you have herpes sores, avoid sex until they are completely healed. This will be less necessary as time goes on and your attacks occur less often.

If you have oral herpes sores, don't have oral-genital or oral-anal sex. Also, remember that if you have herpes sores anywhere, your saliva may be infectious. Don't use saliva as a lubricant during intercourse, or clean your contact lenses with saliva. Wash your hands with soap after touching areas with active sores.

Some of these measures may seem harsh, but nobody wants to spread an infection which can lead to cancer and which at present is incurable. Hopefully, this state of affairs is temporary. Until that time, we must all proceed with caution.

One more note for herpes victims who are sexually active: Don't always assume that what looks like a recurrence of herpes is. Check for syphilis if you see a sore which isn't in the same spot as the primary herpes infection.

Herpes and Pregnancy

An active case of genital herpes can be quite serious during pregnancy and there is no way of getting around that fact. About 50 percent of babies born to women with an active case of herpes develop neonatal herpes. Sixty percent of the time it is fatal to the infant, and if the infant survives there may be lifelong brain damage.

A baby can be protected from infection by a caesarean delivery either before or as soon as possible after the membrane has ruptured. So, a woman who has had attacks of herpes should be tested by her obstetrician at weekly intervals in her ninth month to check for subclinical infection (infection which is present without symptoms).

If you have herpes sores, be careful that your hands are completely clean when you are touching your children on thin membranes such as their eyes, mouths and genital areas. If you have oral sores, refrain from kissing them on those membranes.

7: Nonongococcal Urethritis (NGU)

ITS NAME TELLS YOU what it isn't—it isn't gonorrhea, although for men the symptoms are very similar—both result in an inflammation of the urethra.

It is common, so common that it's supposed to be the most prevalent STD in the United States. The people who study such things say that the average male with NGU tends to be young, unmarried, heterosexual, white and from a middle or higher socio-economic group.

Almost all urethritis seen in college health services and by most private doctors is NGU. Gonorrhea is epidemic, but NGU is thought to be more than twice as common! There's no convenient label for *that* much disease.

There's very little convenient about NGU from a medical standpoint. If not taken care of it can lead to a chronic case of urethritis in men, or it may spread into the prostate or the epididymis, causing widespread infection and both physical and psychological distress.

As with gonorrhea, if the eye is exposed to infectious genital secretions from NGU, inclusion conjuctivitis may develop. This affects children as well as adults. (For a discussion of conjunctivitis, see the section on NGU and pregnancy at the end of this chapter.)

Women sex contacts of men with NGU, who are not treated, may wind up with PID.* And both men and women who engage in rectal intercourse with men who have NGU may develop proctitis, an inflammation of the lining of the rectum.

The foregoing isn't intended to scare anyone, since NGU usually responds well to treatment, but to impress upon you the need to attend to NGU if you think you have it, and to make sure that all your sexual contacts in the month prior to onset of your condition get treated too. The necessity of treating female sex contacts of men with NGU—because they are a frequent source of reinfection and, most important, because they are at risk for PID—is just beginning to be recognized by the medical establishment.

Mode of Transmission

NGU is transmitted during sexual intercourse with a person carrying the organisms that cause the infection—or it can be carried on the hands to the eyes.

It's caused by several different organisms, some of which researchers haven't isolated yet. Luckily, they've identified the two most common organisms—*Chlamydia trachomatis,* which accounts for almost a half of all cases, and *Ureaplasma urealyticum,* which accounts for another quarter of all cases. Both respond to the same treatment. We'll mention some other causes for NGU at the end of this chapter.

Symptoms

Urethritis is an inflammation of the urethra—and we're talking about men here; we'll talk about women in a minute—which causes a burning sensation upon urination and a urethral discharge. The symptoms appear about one to three weeks after exposure to the infection and are usually milder than gonorrhea.

The discharge may be scant, clearish white or look like mucus. It's more obvious first thing in the morning or following a long period without urination. The burning sensation during urination may be mild or even absent; on the other hand, some men may have severe symptoms with a heavy discharge and severe burning during urination. About 10 percent of men with NGU are totally asymptomatic even though they can transmit the pathogens.

And this is where women come in. Until recently NGU was thought of as a not-very-serious problem which some men had. We now know that not only do women carry and transmit the organisms that cause NGU but that those organisms can do much long-term damage to them. Chlamydia can cause PID and cystitis.*

But the situation is very much complicated by the fact that women often don't have any immediate symptoms when chlamydia is present on the cervix. Even on examination there are often no abnormalities of the cervix. On the other hand, the cervix may be inflamed and there may be erosions, pus, or abnormal tissue development which would show up on a Pap smear.

Most women don't keep close tabs on their cervix, especially if they aren't having any discomfort at all (but you can; refer to Appendix A). So, generally, women have to be told by a male sex partner that he has been diagnosed for NGU before they suspect chlamydia.

Often a man who's been successfully treated for gonorrhea—in other words, the gonococci have been eradicated—still will have a discharge and urethritis. This is a form of

NGU called PGU—postgonococcal urethritis—to indicate the fact that it comes after gonorrhea.

The organisms which cause PGU may have been in the urethra all the while, possibly even contracted at the same time, but because the incubation period is longer, the symptoms of PGU appear after the gonorrhea has been cured. Penicillin, most often used to cure gonorrhea, is totally ineffective against the organisms that cause NGU.

Testing for NGU

At this time, there's no test widely available that tests specifically for NGU. A male patient who comes to a doctor or clinic with a burn and a discharge is tested for gonorrhea (the procedure is detailed in the chapter on gonorrhea). If a Gram stain test is performed—this is usually done on the spot immediately—and a culture is done—this takes a little longer, usually two to three days—and both tests prove negative for the gonococcus bacteria, then the doctor diagnoses NGU.

Until the results of the culture come back negative, the patient may be medicated as if he has gonorrhea. So it is quite important for a patient to talk to his doctor or clinic within a week after the initial visit to check the culture results. Because, if he is taking penicillin medication for a nonexistent gonococcal infection, it won't help his *real* nongonococcal infection (whereas some other drugs prescribed for gonorrhea are also effective against NGU).

There are no widely available tests for chlamydia or ureaplasma in women. But an undetected infection may lead to PID. So it's up to a woman to be aware of any signs of NGU in her male partner or to be open to any information he can give her about his health.

If any of your sex partners has a discharge, make sure they get screened for gonorrhea and NGU. And get yourself to a clinic or doctor for medication. Be prepared to say whether your partner has gonorrhea or NGU. If you don't know, you should be treated with tetracycline, which is effective against both diseases.

Treating NGU

If you are receiving treatment for NGU, use ALL the medication prescribed according to the proper schedule. If you stop taking it when the symptoms disappear, the infection may very well come back strong, and next time it will be more difficult to get rid of. By the same token, to prevent relapse, if for no other reason, make sure your sexual partners are treated.

There are several drugs which have been found to be effective against the two most common causes of NGU, chlamydia and ureaplasma, but as yet there's no general agreement as to optimum dosages and length of treatment.

Among the medications are tetracycline, doxycycline, minocycline and erythromycin. If you are taking tetracycline, take it an hour before or two hours after meals and stay away from dairy products; they interfere with absorption. Erythromycin is prescribed for those who are allergic to penicillin-type drugs. It should also be substituted for tetracycline during pregnancy, since tetracycline stains the infant's teeth.

For most people, the condition is cured within three weeks. If it isn't, it's time to go back to the doctor. A different antibiotic may be prescribed or the length of treatment may be increased. The other thing to be considered is whether all your sexual contacts have been treated; otherwise you may be experiencing reinfection.

Avoid alcohol until completely cured, since it may irritate the urethra. Also, until you and your partner(s) are cured, use condoms.

If antibiotics don't clear up the NGU, and if sex partners have been treated so that there is no chance of reinfection, and if you are having many recurrences in rapid sequence over a long period of time (say, six months), it's time to think about other possibilities. There may be foreign bodies, or sores or scar tissue possibly incurred in an earlier bout of NGU or gonorrhea—in the urethra. Discovering these requires intensive investigation by a urologist, a doctor specializing in urological problems. But don't jump into this expensive course without first being absolutely sure that you're not being reinfected by sex partners.

Patients who contract chlamydial infections in their eyes are treated with local antibacterial therapy—chlortetracycline eye ointment—as well as oral antibiotics. Pregnant women, children and those allergic to tetracycline substitute erythromycin or sulfonamide.

NGU and Pregnancy

The most serious effects of chlamydial NGU are reserved for infants born to mothers with chlamydia. These women are also at high risk for PID. In the future, when testing methods are more widely available, pregnant women will probably be screened for chlamydia as they now are for gonorrhea and syphilis. At this point, unfortunately, there isn't much that can be done to avoid the risk entirely.

Among the complications that may develop from chlamydia in newborns is neonatal inclusion conjunctivitis and pneumonia.

Conjunctivitis is an inflammation of the mucus membrane which lines the eyelid and the eyeball. One to two weeks after birth, an infant with chlamydial conjunctivitis will develop a redness and a pus discharge from the eyes. The symptoms are similar to gonococcal conjunctivitis, but the treatments are different. If chlamydial conjunctivitis isn't treated, scarring and blindness may occur.

The spread of chlamydia into the lungs of newborns is the leading cause of pneumonia in infants and can be fatal. Parents of a newborn with chlamydial conjunctivitis or pneumonia should receive a full course of treatment for chlamydia.

8: Nonspecific Proctitis (NSP)

Proctitis means an inflammation of the rectum. When it's called nonspecific it means that all the known causes of proctitis have been ruled out. What remains is a painful condition without a determined cause.

Nonspecific proctitis shares symptoms with several other STDs, including anal gonorrhea,* the enteric STDs,* warts,* syphilis * and herpes.* It also resembles problems that are not transmitted sexually, such as mechanical bowel dysfunctions or hemorrhoids (swollen veins in the rectum).

Mode of Transmission

As its name suggests, researchers haven't yet isolated a pathogen responsible for nonspecific proctitis. The condition is most frequently found in people who are receptors in anal intercourse. The likelihood of the problem increases with the frequency of this activity and the insertion of foreign objects into the rectum. The lining of the anus and rectum may become irritated and therefore less able to ward off infectious agents.

Some medical authorities believe that the frequent combination of oral-genital and anal-genital sexual practices predispose the anorectal area to constant irritation and, therefore, to a variety of infections.

Symptoms

Symptoms of nonspecific proctitis may include:

1. rectal pain and, possibly, rectal discharge
2. pain on defecation
3. burning and stinging
4. blood and/or pus and mucus in the stools
5. mild diarrhea or the desire to defecate but inability to do so
6. a sensation of having a foreign object in the rectum

Testing for Nonspecific Proctitis

This is a diagnosis by exclusion. First, you will need to make sure with the appropriate tests that it's not gonorrhea or syphilis. Then you will need a detailed and sensitive examination. It is critical that you see a doctor whom you are comfortable with and can speak to freely.

The doctor will have to know about your sexual practices. You can provide him/her with a great deal of information that can be helpful. Think about the following before your visit:

1. When do you feel the most pain—during sex? during or after defecation?
2. Is there a discharge?
3. Are there any changes in your bowel habits or in your urinary habits? Have you had any other unusual symp-

toms such as diarrhea, gas, constipation, blood in the stools?
4. Are there any other symptoms, even if they don't seem related?
5. Has the pain been getting worse?
6. Do you use rectal lubricants and what are they? Commercial lubricants may contain alcohol (as do some perfumed oils) or other irritants, or substances you are allergic to. For example, Vicks Vaporub contains camphor, which is an irritant.

The doctor should do a careful examination of the anus, feeling for growths, sores, abscesses, lumps or tears in the lining. An anoscope, which is a small instrument that makes the inside of the anus visible, should be used also. To see farther up into the rectum and colon, it may be necessary to use longer instruments, such as a proctoscope and sigmoidoscope. But these are usually left to a proctologist.

Hemorrhoids are the most common cause of rectal bleeding and should be ruled out first. Another frequent possibility in those who practice anal intercourse is warts. If there are bowel disturbances, one of the enteric STDs is a possibility. A biopsy may be performed.

The range of tests you take will depend largely on what diseases your symptoms most resemble, since these will have to be ruled out before a diagnosis of nonspecific proctitis is given.

Treating Nonspecific Proctitis

Treatment for nonspecific proctitis falls in a gray zone since doctors don't always know what causes it. If no definite cause is found, you may be asked to take a broad spectrum antibiotic. This is a medication, such as tetracycline, that kills many pathogens. Another medication which is sometimes prescribed to suppress inflammation is Azulfidine® (salicylazosulfapyridine). But it can have severe side effects and should never be used by pregnant women, asthmatics and those with kidney, liver or blood disorders. It should be used with extreme caution.

Sometimes, nonspecific proctitis resolves itself without treatment.

To relieve immediate discomfort, a doctor may prescribe topical steroids or steroid enemas. But the enteric parasites must be ruled out first, since steroids foster their increase.

Also, try sitting in a hot sitz bath. The heat increases circulation, relieves pain and lessens rectal spasms.

9: Pelvic Inflammatory Disease (PID)

PID IS A CATCH-ALL NAME which refers to infection in any of the organs of a woman's pelvic cavity (see illustrations on pp. 5–6). Once an organ is infected, the infection is easily spread to the other organs in the pelvic cavity. Unless it is treated.

Over a quarter of a million women in the United States develop gonococcal PID yearly. At least an equal number, and probably more, develop PID which is not caused by the gonococcus bacteria. But those cases are not so closely monitored by federal authorities, who concentrate on gonorrhea, so it's hard to get a clear picture.

PID is acknowledged as a leading cause of sterility in women but it's not yet being systematically screened for. While public health clinics and women's health facilities are aware of the problem, on the whole it's up to the individual woman to suspect PID early enough and to make sure she gets proper diagnosis and treatment.

PID and the IUD

One important thing every woman can do to lessen her chances of getting PID is to *use any form of birth control other than the IUD.* Studies have shown repeatedly that women who use an IUD have a two- to nine-fold greater incidence of PID than nonusers. The reason for this seems to be that the IUD dislodges the protective mucous plug in the opening of the cervix (which is known as the os) and so diminishes its normal ability to combat bacteria.

PID in IUD wearers is even higher in women who've never been pregnant. One study found that IUD users who were never pregnant had a four-fold greater incidence of PID than previously pregnant women.

If you think this sounds like a harsh diatribe against the IUD, nothing can be harsh enough as far as we're concerned. The IUD is thought to encourage all kinds of infection, its pull-string acting as a conductor into a woman's body. If you want the choice to give birth in the future, there are other forms of birth control that are just as effective, completely safe and even useful in preventing STDs.

Mode of Transmission

The first time a woman has an attack of PID, it may seem to have struck out of nowhere, without any clear warning. Despite the impression, it would be theoretically possible in most cases to trace it back—and it might well be a while back—to a man who, symptomatic or not, had a case of gonorrhea ° or chlamydial nongonococcal urethritis (NGU).°

The pathogens enter through the vagina during intercourse and make their way up to the cervix. Often they are stopped there by the body's own defense mechanisms. Or, if the pathogen is gonococcal, the woman may develop cervical gonorrhea; if it's detected it can be dealt with successfully at that stage.

Or—and here's the problem—the pathogens may slip

through the cervical os and into the uterus and the fallopian tubes.

In these organs, the bacteria attach themselves to the cells of the mucous linings and destroy them. This results in production of tubal pus. If the pus spills over into the pelvic cavity (the peritoneum), the bacteria will also attack the lining of the abdomen and pelvis.

Several factors have been named which seem to increase the chances that the pathogens will spread beyond the cervix. We've already talked about the IUD. Changes connected with the menstrual cycle also play a role. At least it seems that at the onset of menstruation, the mucous plug which usually covers the os disappears, allowing gonococci free access to points north. In addition, the menstrual blood nourishes the bacteria and acts as its transport system as the blood is recycled through the reproductive system.

Once you have had any kind of PID, you are more likely to get it again. Apparently, damage to the fallopian tubes impairs normal host defense mechanisms, making you more susceptible to infection. With each recurrence, scar tissue accumulates in the fallopian tubes and the chances of pelvic pain, ectopic pregnancy and sterility increase.

Symptoms

The most constant symptom of PID is pain in the pelvic region. This becomes worse over time as the infection progresses, but can also be temporarily heightened by any sort of excessive motion, including intercourse. The way pelvic pain is perceived is a very individual matter, but typically it occurs on both sides of the lower abdomen. In the early stages, it may be possible to ignore it and, unfortunately, many women do. Later on, however, the pain may become so severe that any movement is impossible.

Other symptoms which may or may not accompany the pain include:

1. increased menstrual cramps
2. pain during intercourse
3. pain during ovulation
4. bleeding outside of—or profusely during—menstruation
5. nausea, loss of appetite and vomiting
6. chills and fever
7. a vaginal discharge
8. burning during urination
9. tenderness around the liver if the infection has spread.

Testing for PID

Pain in the pelvis can indicate a whole range of problems. For example, it may signal acute appendicitis, ruptured ovarian cysts, a tubal (ectopic) pregnancy, a kidney infection or a spontaneous abortion caused by pathogenic micro-organisms or other toxins. In all cases, an immediate medical visit is in order. If you've been using an IUD, have it removed.

Whenever there is pelvic pain, there is need for a bimanual pelvic examination to locate the source of the pain. In fact, any internal examination for women, even the most routine one, should include a bimanual to check for incipient tenderness. The bimanual is simple and doesn't demand any sophisticated instruments, just two hands.

What should happen is that the person performing the examination inserts two fingers of one hand into the vagina while using the other hand on the outside to press down on different areas of the abdominal and pelvic cavities. The fingers inside move systematically from one site to the other while the fingers above press down on the same sites. This doesn't have to be time-consuming or uncomfortable. However, if you have a severe case of PID, it won't be easy.

To determine whether the cause of PID is gonococcal or nongonococcal, specimens are usually taken from the cervix and the anus and cultured. A blood test is also done.

Treating PID

In any case, before the doctor knows whether you have gonococcal or nongonococcal PID, you'll receive the treatment for gonorrhea which, as described in that chapter, is usually an injection of procaine penicillin to each of the buttocks.

Then you'll follow up with ampicillin (if allergic, then tetracycline) taken in doses of 500 mg. four times a day. If you are taking tetracycline, take it at least an hour before or two hours after meals and avoid dairy products because they interfere with absorption.

The medication is extremely important, but it is only half of the treatment needed for PID. It's essential that a woman with PID give herself time for rest and recuperation. Stay in bed and allow the tissues to mend. Eat simply and well. Avoid intercourse entirely. Most important, even when you think you've healed entirely, *don't sleep with a partner who hasn't been tested for gonorrhea and NGU, even if he's asymptomatic.* Studies show that a high percentage of women with PID have male sex partners with asymptomatic gonorrhea.

See your doctor to make sure you are completely well again. If you are not, your infection may be caused by a resistant pathogen and you will need to try alternative medications. Further examination may be necessary. Sometimes in these cases, a hospital stay is necessary.

Hospitalization is frequently advised when a woman is

pregnant, has a high fever, is found to have pelvic abscesses or when oral medication is causing nausea and vomiting (so that medication must be given intravenously). In the hospital, more sophisticated instruments such as the laparoscope are used to examine the peritoneal cavity. Another process, called culdocentesis, is usually performed to attempt to identify the pathogen definitively. A needle is inserted into the abdomen and fluid is aspirated out, cultured and examined.

10: Scabies

SCABIES IS OFTEN CONFUSED with allergic reactions, insect bites, crabs *, syphilis *, eczema and a variety of other skin conditions. If you develop an itch on the surface of your skin at about the same time members of your family and/or close friends do, there's a good chance you all have scabies. Anyone can get it, anyone can spread it and anyone can get rid of it by following the simple instructions we'll outline later on in this chapter.

Mode of Transmission

The *Sarcoptes scabiei* is a tiny mite, barely visible to the naked eye, which makes its home in skin. It moves quickly and easily among people. As with some of the other sexually transmissible diseases, it is not dependent on sexual encounters for its mobility, but the chances of becoming a host to the mite do rise as your level of sexual activity with different partners rises.

Sarcoptes scabiei is nicknamed "itch mite" for its most striking quality. The itch is a reaction to the mite. The female burrows through the skin and starts laying eggs at the rate of two to three a day. These eggs hatch in three to four days and become adults in about ten days.

The Symptoms

There are two ways of suspecting that your itch may be a scabies itch: The scabies itch is a shared one (friends and family members will probably be experiencing it too); and it is more severe at night.

For a person who has never had scabies before, it may take a month or longer after the female burrows through the skin for the reaction to occur. During this time it is possible to spread the infection even though you are not aware you have it. A person who has had scabies will show symptoms sooner, as soon as a day after reinfection.

There is another physical symptom: The burrows the mites make manifest themselves to the naked eye as ridges or streaks. They are most common between the fingers; inside the wrists or elbows; and in the folds of the upper arm. Also, you may see them around the nipples; on the belly; the folds of the buttocks; the penis; feet and ankles; and around the waist. (In adults, they are never above the neck.) Of course, they itch.

If you look at the ridges with a magnifying glass, you'll perhaps recognize the burrow which the mite makes. It looks like a short, dirty, wavy line. There may be a small red bump along the burrow which contains the mite. But these bumps are often broken due to scratching and the burrow may be difficult to see.

Frequent bathing, although it may relieve the itching, also makes scabies difficult to detect. Individual mites on the surface of the skin are washed away and the burrows and lesions are much less visible. But soap and water alone will not remove the mites which are under the skin and it won't cure the infestation. Medication is necessary.

Testing for Scabies

If you suspect you have scabies—either because you've been intimate with someone who has scabies, or because you have an itch which is more intense at night and/or is shared by intimates—you should speak to a doctor.

Sometimes a doctor will prescribe medication on the basis of symptoms alone. Since the medication is cheap and reasonably safe, s/he may think it's worth trying this first to see whether it works.

Doctors can test for scabies by examining scrapings taken from a burrow which has not been scratched open by the patient. The burrow is scraped with a needle or a blade and the scraping is examined under a microscope for the mite, her eggs or fecal pellets.

Treating Scabies

First and foremost—try not to scratch! Excessive scratching may lead to a bacterial infection. And then if that's not treated, you might end up with a systemic bacterial infection, which is a lot more serious than scabies.

The doctor will probably prescribe lindane cream or lotion, commonly sold as Kwell® or Gamene.® It's a prescription drug which costs only a few dollars a bottle, is easy to use and highly effective.

Lindane is applied over the entire body, excluding the face, to treat scabies. You take a warm soap and water bath, or shower, and towel dry gently. Then apply the cream or lotion working from the neck downwards and paying special attention to the hands—especially between the fingers—and the wrists, the feet, between the toes, the ankles, the creases and folds of the neck, the groin, legs, armpits and beneath the breasts. Apply thinly and thoroughly, but avoid the eyes and mucous membranes. Leave it on for twenty-four hours before washing.

All items of clothing, bed linens and towels which you've used should be washed and dried by machine on a hot cycle or dry-cleaned.

Anybody you've been in intimate contact with should be treated simultaneously, even if they don't have symptoms.

A second application of lindane a week after the first may be recommended to destroy recently hatched mites, since the medication may not destroy all the mites' eggs. But don't use lindane more often than necessary, since it is absorbed by the body and can cause skin inflammation.

Infants, young children and pregnant women should not be treated with lindane, since it is absorbed through the skin and into the bloodstream.

An alternative to lindane, prescribed for pregnant women, is crotamiton, sold by prescription as Eurax.® It is a cream that is massaged into the skin from the neck downward and reapplied after twenty-four hours. As with lindane, do your laundry and make sure your intimate contacts are treated.

The itch and symptoms of scabies may not disappear for several weeks after treatment. This is because the hypersensitive reaction of the skin to the mite doesn't clear up as soon as the mites are destroyed. Some people don't understand this and become very anxious when the itch persists. Anxiety and scratching can prolong post-treatment itching. And people who are prone to allergies may have severe post-treatment itching.

Be patient. If you've used the medicine as directed and

taken care of the possible sources of reinfestation, the treatment will be effective. You may want to ask your doctor about antihistamines or a lotion to soothe the itching. If a bacterial infection sets in, antibiotics are in order.

Scabies in Infants and Young Children

Scabies in infants and young children is frequently misdiagnosed. The infestation is usually not suspected. Also, the characteristic burrows are frequently absent and the distribution of the rash isn't typical.

The skin may be highly inflamed, red and itchy, with small, pimple-like, fluid-filled sacs that ooze and dry up to form crusty scabs. They may be seen on the head of an infant, the neck, the palms of the hands and the soles of the feet.

The preferred treatment for scabies in young children and infants is sulfur ointment. The medication is applied three nights in a row. Individuals may bathe before reapplying the medication. Sulfur is messy, smelly and stains. But it doesn't carry any of the possible problems of lindane.

Be sure to take all the precautions against reinfestation described in TREATING SCABIES above.

11: Syphilis

AMONG STDs, SYPHILIS is a special case. It can easily be detected, treated and cured. *But* if it's not, it can become a dread disease. It is the oldest recognized STD and should be extinct by now, given the understanding and techniques we have to deal with it. But, since the late '50s, it's woven a wavy path upward to the stars.

These days, the ratio of men who catch syphilis to women is three to one. Fifty percent of all men who get it have same-sex partners. This makes syphilis a major problem for the gay male population.

If you have been in contact with someone who has syphilis: Most important, resist becoming anxious about it. But do something immediately. With treatment, it can be prevented in the incubation period. But if syphilis slips by unnoticed, it may reappear many years later in the heart, brain or some other organ. If you are sexually active, have your blood checked regularly, at least every six months.

If you are even at the slightest risk for contracting syphilis, read on. It's worth your while for you to familiarize yourself with the technical information we're going to provide in this chapter. And if you've ever had syphilis in the past, there's some important information for you about blood tests.

Mode of Transmission

Syphilis is contracted during sexual contact with someone who is in an infectious stage of the disease. The infection is spread from open sores or rashes which are filled with spiral shaped bacteria called *Treponema pallidum.* They are able to penetrate the thin membranes which line the genitals, the anus and the mouth.

If the sores are inside the anus or vagina, they won't be visible, but if you do see a sore on yourself or a sex partner, don't have sex until it's checked out. Or at least use a condom until test results come in.

Symptoms

The symptoms of syphilis can be divided into four stages: primary and secondary stages, during which the disease is highly infectious; and latent and late stages.

THE PRIMARY STAGE The signature of primary syphilis is a sore, also called a chancre or a lesion. There is usually just one, but there can be more. It can appear wherever there is a break on the skin, but it most frequently occurs on the mucous membrane linings of the labia, penis, or the mouth. It may be inside the anus, the vagina or the urethra and therefore invisible to ordinary inspection. (A woman can check for sores on her cervix or vagina with the use of a speculum; refer to Appendix A.)

The chancre marks the spot where the syphilis bacteria, *Treponema pallidum,* first enters the body, traveling directly from an open sore on somebody else's body. Syphilis enters the bloodstream a few hours after the treponeme enters the body, but it won't become immediately apparent, and a test at this point won't pick it up. It will take anywhere from ten to ninety days for the chancre to appear.

At first it will be a hard bump and then it will burst and run for awhile and then become crusty. This is all usually painless. There will also be a swollen gland in the immediate vicinity. The whole process takes about two to three weeks and heals without a sign after four to six weeks, whether or not the syphilis is treated.

It's easy to miss a syphilitic sore, especially if it's located inside the mouth, vagina or anus. Even when it is right on the penis, it can be mistaken for a zipper cut, friction burn or an ingrown hair. If there's any chance that a sore might be syphilitic, get it tested. (If you engage in anal intercourse, be sure to tell your doctor to check for anal chancres.) If it is syphilis, all your contacts for the last three months must be tested immediately.

THE SECONDARY STAGE If you've missed the chancre in the primary stage, there are some symptoms which may occur a little later (usually a few months after the syphilis is contracted and about a month after the primary stage ends).

1. Rashes—either flat, or raised and reddish, usually not itchy; may occur anywhere on the body; or
   —a symmetrical rash that occurs simultaneously on the palms of the hands and the soles of the feet
2. Sores in the mouth or on the genitals
3. Loss of patches of hair on the scalp, eyelashes or eyebrows

4. Cracks in the folds of the mouth or nose
5. Moist, highly infectious wart-like lesions in the ano-genital region
6. Swollen glands throughout the body
7. Fever and a general feeling of poor health
8. Black people may get large round or half-moon shaped sores on their faces

Some people show several of these symptoms and others show none; they may be severe and they may be mild. Everyone reacts differently during secondary syphilis.

The symptoms will go away after a few weeks (two to six) with or without treatment. Although some untreated people experience a relapse of the secondary stage at some point during the next two years, most enter the latent stage and no longer show signs of syphilis.

If you discover that you have secondary syphilis, you must notify all your sexual contacts as far back as six months.

THE LATENT STAGE Syphilis left untreated proceeds into the latent stage. During this time there are no symptoms and the disease can't be spread to other people. The latent stage may last the rest of an infected person's life. It will at least last a few years. If a blood test for syphilis is taken during this period, it will show positive, and the disease will be treated. All of your sex partners during the past year should be contacted and tested.

THE LATE STAGE Syphilis can kill. If many years elapse and a person still hasn't received treatment, complications can occur involving the cardiovascular and central nervous systems. Irreversible tissue damage can occur anywhere on or in the body.

Testing for Syphilis

Syphilis testing is done routinely and usually free of charge in public health clinics. A clinic may be the best bet for syphilis treatment on several counts: All clinics have the special darkfield microscopes for immediate identification of the treponeme; clinic workers are experienced at interpreting the blood tests; they're free and syphilis can get very expensive if treated by a private doctor; and there is always a public health advisor on the premises to answer any questions you may have (we'll talk more about public health advisors in the section on treatment).

Syphilis tests need a bit of explaining but they are important to understand. If you have a suspicious sore or rash, you should have it tested. Don't wash or apply antiseptic solutions to it before testing; this will make the treponemes hard to detect.

The darkfield examination detects treponemes from syphilitic sores (unless the sore is in the mouth, in which case it's ineffective). The sore will be scraped and then pinched until a drop of clear fluid can be put onto a slide; then it's examined under a darkfield microscope, which only allows a little bit of light to enter from the side. If the treponeme is present, it will pick up the light and appear as a small whirling spiral or corkscrew.

If the darkfield is positive, you will receive immediate treatment. Even if the results are negative, you should have a blood test for syphilis. If that is negative, repeat it in a few weeks to be absolutely sure.

Blood tests are generally given to determine the stage of the syphilis infection. Also, if you have a suspicious sore in your mouth, this is the only way to find out whether it's syphilitic.

There are several different blood tests for syphilis; they

all measure the amount of antibody reaction to the treponemal bacteria which cause syphilis. There are two classes of antibodies measured: antibodies which react only to syphilitic treponemes and other antibodies which are less specific.

The blood tests which measure only the antibodies specific to syphilis are called the treponemal tests. The less specific tests are called nontreponemal. The latter are the most commonly used because they are inexpensive and easy to perform. In all cases, be sure not to take any antibiotics before taking the blood test.

The VDRL (which stands for Venereal Disease Research Laboratory) is a common nontreponemal test. It's usually performed at public health clinics free or at private laboratories for about $5.

If your VDRL is positive, it means that antibodies in your blood have reacted to the addition of an antigen. And if it is positive, the lab technician will go on to measure the amount of antibody reaction by diluting the blood until no reactions occur. The last dilution which gives a positive reaction is called the titer. The more antibodies you have, the more you have to dilute the blood; the more you have to dilute the blood, the higher the titer is.

The titer rises during the infectious stages of the disease. During the latent stage of untreated syphilis, the titer is low but doesn't disappear. At this time the only way to know that a person has syphilis is through a blood test. If reinfection or relapse occurs, the titer begins to climb again.

A positive VDRL can also be triggered by hepatitis, mononucleosis, a recent smallpox vaccination, narcotic addiction, a systemic illness, old age and nothing at all to name a few. This is called a false positive reaction.

But a positive treponemal test usually means one thing—syphilis. The main exceptions are yaws, bejel and pinta, all diseases caused by a related treponeme and which are common among people from the tropics or the Caribbean area. If you've had any of these diseases, you should mention it when you're tested for syphilis.

Specific treponemal tests such as the FTA (Fluorescent Treponemal Antibody Absorption) or HA (Hemagglutination) are difficult to perform, more costly and time-consuming. Therefore, they should only be administered when there is reason to suspect that the positive reaction to the VDRL or other nontreponemal test has been triggered by something other than syphilis.

Treating Syphilis

Let's face it: All blood tests that are positive for syphilis are reported to the local public health officials. It's a law and laboratories won't risk their licenses by withholding the information. But these records are strictly confidential and can't even be subpoenaed in a court of law. So there's no reason to go to a private doctor just for privacy's sake.

If you are diagnosed as having syphilis, whether you're at a private doctor or a clinic, you can speak to a public health advisor. They're available everywhere in the United States. They specialize in syphilis and they have a lot of time to spend with you, providing helpful information and answering any questions you may have.

The first thing to know is that primary, secondary and latent syphilis can be nipped in the bud with penicillin. You may receive one or several large doses of special long-acting penicillin injections. There may be some soreness at the injection site; this will pass, but walking or a hot bath may help. For those allergic to penicillin, a long course of tetracycline is prescribed. Pregnant women who are allergic to penicillin are treated with erythromycin.

If you are being treated for early infectious syphilis, about forty-eight hours after receiving the penicillin injection, you are no longer infectious. But you are quite likely to get what is known as a Herxheimer reaction a few hours after the injection. It feels like you've come down with the flu—fever; chills; headache; general ill health. If you have a rash, it might get temporarily worse. Take an aspirin and spend the day in bed. You'll be fine tomorrow.

During the next year, it's necessary to have a blood test every three months to monitor your recovery. The titer should be dropping consistently. During the second year, it's OK to decrease your visits to the doctor by 50 percent, that is once every six months. VDRL titers of people treated during the primary stage of syphilis usually return to negative within a year after treatment. If treatment began in the secondary stage, it will take a bit longer, about eighteen months.

In a very small percentage of cases the titer drops but never returns to negative even though the patient has been cured of syphilis. This is called serofast. If you are serofast, you will know if you are reinfected when your titer rises or when you see signs of the infection. Otherwise there's no reason to subject yourself to expensive treatment again and again.

It is extremely important for anybody who has or had syphilis to understand titers, but it is especially important for somebody who is serofast. Whenever a serofast person has a VDRL, whether for a marriage license, hospital admission, new employment or a professional license, there will be a positive reaction. A note from your physician stating that you've been adequately treated and aren't infectious may be required. Legally you cannot be denied employment if you've had syphilis in the past and were treated properly.

If you change doctors, it's a good idea to inform him/her about your past history and, if you are serofast, to tell your doctor what your titer usually is. Everyone with syphilis should keep his/her own records of tests, with dates, results and treatments.

Syphilis and Pregnancy

If syphilis is contracted in pregnancy and remains untreated, the chances that it will affect the fetus are very high. In most instances the infant will be stillborn or have congenital malformations.

After the fourth month of pregnancy, treponemes are able to pass through the placenta of a pregnant woman who has syphilis. If syphilis is detected before the fifth month of pregnancy and treated, the deformities of congenital syphilis probably won't occur. All pregnant women should be tested for syphilis at least twice: at the onset of pregnancy and toward the end.

If you've had syphilis and have been adequately treated for it before becoming pregnant, it poses no risk to the baby. Also, an untreated case of syphilis that was contracted long before pregnancy is less likely to affect the baby.

But the importance of early and adequate prenatal care cannot be overemphasized. It's important insurance against the undeserved punishment of congenital syphilis.

12: Vaginitis

VAGINITIS LITERALLY means inflammation of the vagina. "Inflammation" is characterized by heat, redness, swelling and pain. For most women, the obvious characteristic of vaginitis is the itch.

If you have a vagina, at one time or another you're bound to have an itch. It isn't always sexually transmitted; in fact the most common form of vaginitis, candidiasis, is brought on by organisms normally found in a woman's genital tract. (The same organisms that cause vaginitis may also cause problems for men; these are discussed below.)

A Key to the Subchapters

We've divided this chapter into three sections based on the cause of the vaginitis:

The time it takes you to seek treatment for vaginitis will probably depend partly on the severity of the itch, partly on your capacity to withstand discomfort. But you should definitely not ignore it. To treat it effectively, it's important to understand a few things about:

1. the three different causes
2. the probability of reinfection from a male sex partner.

What may feel like vaginitis could be another of the STDs (especially gonorrhea *) which is more dangerous to your health. Or you may have vaginitis and gonorrhea simultaneously; this is a fairly frequent occurrence. So be sure to get tested for gonorrhea when you're seen for vaginitis, since treatment for vaginitis won't cure gonorrhea or prevent the complications of gonorrhea.

In order to distinguish between the three forms of vaginitis, it is essential that your doctor do a wet mount smear test or at least a culture and a Pap smear. These infections can't be identified on the basis of signs and symptoms alone. Don't douche before going to the doctor because it interferes with the laboratory tests.

In the three subchapters, for each of the diseases, we're going to talk about its mode of transmission, its symptoms, the medical means of identifying it, its treatment and how—if at all—it affects pregnancy. It would be helpful, both for the doctor and yourself, if you did a self-examination so you could be more explicit about your problem (see Appendix A).

Candidiasis

Mode of Transmission

Candida albicans is a yeast-like fungus which normally lives in the mouth, gastrointestinal tract, rectum and vagina. It is only when there is an overgrowth of the organism that it becomes a problem.

Overgrowth occurs frequently in several situations. The incidence in pregnant women for example is estimated to be ten to twenty times higher. Women who are predisposed to diabetes, post-menopausal or eating a diet high in sugar and starch are more likely to get it. Certain drugs, including oral contraceptives, antibiotics, metronidazole (Flagyl®), steroids, and immunosuppressive drugs, may also cause overgrowth. Men who have candidiasis usually get it from women. *C. albicans* is often found in the urethra of male sex partners of women with candidiasis.

Symptoms

In women:
1. The itch—it usually begins right before menstruation.
2. A discharge, which may be thin and watery, but is usually thick and white and sometimes described as "cottage cheese." It tends to smell yeasty.
3. Pain, possibly during intercourse, or burning during urination.
4. Self-examination may reveal that the vulva is swollen and red. White patches may be seen on the vulva and vagina.

In men:
1. Mild burning during urination or itching of the penis.
2. Dry, glazed redness at the head of the penis.
3. Possibly small, irregularly shaped eroded bumps and dispersed little sacs containing white cheesey matter under or around the head of the penis or over the entire penis or scrotum.

Testing for Candidiasis

The main point of a doctor's diagnosis is to differentiate candidiasis from other forms of vaginitis. Make sure not to douche, use drugs or apply a topical cream before your visit to the doctor, since they may mask the organism in lab tests.

A specimen of your discharge will be examined under a microscope for a large number of active yeast cells. Your discharge may also be cultured, both for yeast and gonorrhea. If cultures are done, call up in a few days to get the results.

Treating Candidiasis

There are three commonly prescribed medications for candidiasis. They are: nystatin, which comes in cream and suppository form; miconazole cream; and clotrimazole vaginal tablets or cream. They are all inserted into the vagina once or twice daily for a week or two, and are usually quite effective. But they may be a little messy; you can avoid this by using sanitary mini-pads.

Medical authorities haven't yet decided whether treating asymptomatic male partners is necessary. But, if you have a recurrent infection, it's worth trying. The treatment for the male, which your doctor can prescribe, is nystatin, miconazole or clotrimazole cream applied directly to the penis several times a day. While you and/or your partner are undergoing treatment, it's best to use a condom.

A number of women have recurrent candidiasis. If you are one of these, you may be interested in the experience of several women who say that they have changed the acidity level of their vaginas and discouraged the growth of the fungus by increasing their intake of plain yogurt, or by adding acidophilus culture—sold in health food stores in powder or tablet, and liquid forms—to their diets. Medical treatment for recurrent candidiasis is long-term anti-fungal medication.

Things to avoid are an excessive amount of starchy and sweet food; nylon underwear; pantyhose; tight pants; vaginal deodorants and bubble baths. Always wipe from front to back after using the toilet.

Candidiasis and Pregnant Women

Because miconazole cream (Monistat®) is absorbed through the vagina, most physicians won't prescribe it during the first three months of pregnancy. They'll prescribe a form of nystatin instead.

Infants delivered through the birth canal of mothers with candidiasis have a three-fold greater chance of developing a fungus infection in their mouth which is called "thrush," or on their skin, usually in the diaper area.

Trichomoniasis

Mode of Transmission

Trichomoniasis has reached epidemic proportions in the United States. Although it's usually sexually transmitted, *Trichomonas vaginalis*, a pear-shaped parasite which moves by means of its flagella, can survive on wet objects such as washcloths, sponges or douching equipment for several hours. It may in rare instances be transmitted that way. Some researchers have also reported occasional spread of the infection from mothers to their female infants during childcare. Men are often asymptomatic carriers, harboring the parasite in the penis and transferring it to women during sexual intercourse. Women can also be asymptomatic.

In order to cure trichomoniasis, it is absolutely necessary to treat sexual contacts. The drug that's usually administered is a strong one with some undesirable side effects, so that avoiding reinfection is very important.

Symptoms

In women:

1. The itch—frequently noticeable during or immediately following menstruation.
2. The discharge—may range from thin and slight to heavy, frothy, greenish-yellow and bad-smelling.
3. Burning possibly during urination, and a desire to urinate frequently (could also be cystitis *).
4. Vaginal soreness and pain on intercourse sometimes.
5. The glands in the genital region may be swollen.
6. Occasionally, dull lower abdominal pain (this may be due to a concurrent infection such as gonorrhea * or PID *).
7. On self-examination with a speculum, you will see a green-yellow, frothy discharge on the vaginal walls. The cervix and upper vagina may have a red speckled appearance, known as "strawberry cervix."

In men: Men are almost always asymptomatic, but may notice a mild itch; redness of the penis; discomfort during urination; or pain during intercourse; and a slight urethral discharge. Uncircumcised men may notice a discharge from under the foreskin. For a very few men, discharge and burning are more severe.

Testing for Trichomoniasis

As in candidiasis, the object of the lab test is to rule out the two other forms of vaginitis and simultaneously to check for gonorrhea. Trichomonads can be relatively easily identified on a Gram-stained smear or a wet mount in a doctor's office. Also the Pap smear, usually done to screen women for abnormal cell growths on the cervix, will also turn up trichomonads, but not as well as the Gram stain or wet mount, the usual tests.

To find out if a man has trichomonads in his urethra, a smear test is usually not sufficient, since urination washes out the trichomonads making the infection difficult to detect. Instead, a bit of discharge is cultured; it's recommended that the sample is taken before passing the first urine in the morning.

However, if you're a woman being treated for trichomoniasis, your doctor can prescribe treatment for your sex partner without examining him personally. There's very little point in being treated unless he also receives treatment, since the chance of reinfection is so great.

Treating Trichomoniasis

The medicine most often prescribed for trichomoniasis—metronidazole, which usually sells under the brand name Flagyl®—has received a bit of notoriety in recent years. It's been found to cause malignant tumors and physical defects in the offspring of laboratory animals. However, the animals were administered high doses of the drug for long periods of time. At this point there is no evidence of that sort of damage to humans. Its use is a matter of personal judgment.

On the other hand, women who are pregnant or nursing definitely shouldn't take Flagyl.® Try to deal with the infection topically. The possibilities include povidine-iodine douches or douching with vinegar and water or using vaginal suppositories. Trichomoniasis is uncomfortable, but it doesn't appear to be associated with any serious maternal or fetal abnormalities.

In the past, metronidazole was prescribed three times a day for a week, but recent studies show that a single low dose taken orally, both by a woman and her regular sex partner(s), is equally effective.

If you are taking it, avoid drinking alcoholic beverages. They can cause cramps, nausea, vomiting, dizziness and headaches. And, if you are prone to candidiasis, you might want to take some preventative steps: i.e., eat a lot of yogurt and/or acidophilus; ask your doctor for medication for candidiasis.

Use condoms until all partners are fully treated and the infection has been cured.

Nonspecific Vaginitis (NSV)

Mode of Transmission

The principal cause of bacterial vaginitis is *Gardnerella vaginalis* (also called *Haemophilus vaginalis* or *Corynebacterium vaginale)*. There may be other bacterial causes, but they are not yet well understood. At least, and luckily, they can all be treated in basically the same way.

Symptoms

In women:

1. The itch—much milder than with trich or candidiasis. It doesn't seem related to the menstrual cycle.
2. A disagreeable fishy odor—the most distinguishing characteristic.
3. A slight, grayish discharge.
4. Possibly a mild, burning sensation.

5. Self-examination may turn up a homogeneous, relatively thin, sometimes frothy, gray-white discharge which sticks uniformly to the vaginal wall and looks like "flour paste." The vulva may be slightly red and there may be pinpoint dots on the vaginal walls.

In men: Men don't seem to develop symptoms. But it is thought that they can carry the bacteria and reinfect women sex partners if they aren't treated simultaneously.

Testing for NSV

If a woman visits her doctor with a case of vaginitis and the smear test doesn't turn up either *C. albicans* or *T. vaginalis,* s/he will probably assume the patient has NSV.

Treating NSV

The most commonly prescribed treatment for NSV is ampicillin. Since the treatment can mask gonorrhea or syphilis, but not cure either of them, it's imperative to be tested for those two STDs before beginning treatment for NSV.

Another possible treatment is with metronidazole. As we mentioned in the section on trichomoniasis, there are some facts which should be considered before taking it. And if you are pregnant or nursing, you shouldn't take it at all.

Some doctors prescribe sulfonamide-containing creams when a specific pathogen hasn't been isolated. But there is no evidence that they are effective.

13: Warts

ANOGENITAL WARTS, officially known as condylomata acuminata, are on the increase, having more than doubled in reported incidence in recent years. The warmth and moisture in the genital area and anus are extremely conducive to their growth and spread. They are relatively easy to deal with and only very rarely have serious complications, but can be irritating nonetheless.

Mode of Transmission

Warts are thought to result when the papova virus invades the skin of the genitalia or anus. Not everyone is susceptible but it's been estimated that about 60 percent of the sexual partners of infected persons contract warts. If you've contracted warts once, you're one of those who's susceptible and should be careful to make sure that your sexual partners don't have them, or, if they do, that you use barrier prevention.

Warts are highly infectious, even when they are still in the incubation stage and not yet visible or detectable. So there is a possibility of contracting warts even if your partner shows no sign of a wart. Spreading can be stymied considerably if sexual partners use barrier prevention during sex when one of the partners has warts.

Also, if you contract warts, it's important to prevent reinfection by making sure your partners don't have them, or are treating them also. This may mean a doctor's visit, since an anoscope is needed to detect warts in the anus and a special examination is needed to detect warts on the cervix. The incubation period is so long—anywhere from six weeks to six months—that your partner may develop warts after you've been cured and reinfect you.

Symptoms

Warts are skin growths which can:

1. look stem-like, branch-like or cauliflower-like; and
2. may be whitish, grayish, yellowish or pinkish; and
3. may multiply or enlarge to form clusters; and
4. grow anywhere on the skin of the genitals, anus or even mouth and throat, but occur most commonly at and around the following sites:

THE PENIS The virus often invades the skin of the penis in the area subject to pressure during intercourse. This is most common in uncircumcised men. The warts may also occur inside the urethra and even spread into the bladder, but this is rare.

FEMALE GENITALIA Warts occur most commonly on the outer genital area, but may also grow inside the vagina or on the cervix.

THE ANUS Anal warts are most often found in people who engage in rectal intercourse. In women, warts are sometimes spread from the genitals to the perineum to the anus.

Because anal warts sometimes bleed during a bowel movement or anal intercourse, they can be mistaken for hemorrhoids. If you experience anal bleeding and your sexual practices include rectal intercourse, tell your doctor. This will prevent misdiagnosis.

Testing for Warts

Usually warts are quite easily identified by appearance. However there are a few other conditions which resemble them, so it's important for a doctor to do certain tests such as a blood test for syphilis to rule out other possibilities.

Sometimes a biopsy is done. A small piece of skin tissue is removed and examined under a microscope to check for any unusual cell growth. This is to rule out the possibility that the growth is malignant and to make a more accurate identification. Since one of the common treatments for warts, podophyllin, can alter the appearance of the cells, it should not be applied before biopsy.

Biopsy and further investigation is especially necessary if there are unusual symptoms such as pain, if the lesions are ulcerated (open sores) or if there is a serum-blood discharge. But this is relatively rare.

Treating Warts

Don't wait for a wart to disappear spontaneously because usually it won't. They tend to multiply, and then removal becomes complicated and painful. Even when you do have the wart removed immediately, there is a good chance you will have to repeat the treatment again within the year because they tend to grow back. This is annoying to say the least, but persistence will be rewarded in the end. Recurrences of warts that have been removed are less frequent after the first year.

There are many different treatments for warts. The doctor will prescribe one, or more than one in combination, depending on the individual case. You should ask about:

1. the duration of the treatment
2. the amount of discomfort involved
3. the possibility of scarring
4. the relative expense of the treatment

Podophyllin is the most commonly used medication at the moment for ano-genital warts. There are two big exceptions: It cannot be used on pregnant women and it is not effective for hardened warts.

Podophyllin is applied in a doctor's office or clinic once or twice a week until the warts clear up. You must wash the podophyllin off four to six hours after application. If the medication is left on too long, it may cause burning and painful swelling.

If the wart hasn't cleared up after about a month, an alternative treatment should be tried. There have been many instances of people who have spent inordinate amounts of time and money on podophyllin treatments without getting results.

Some doctors prefer to apply acid, carbon dioxide snow or liquid nitrogen to the warts. This method involves fewer visits to the doctor's office and is therefore less expensive, but there is likely to be some scarring. Also some pain—a local anesthetic is usually administered.

Surgery and electrodessication are usually reserved for warts that are very large or fail to respond to other treatments, or that occur in pregnant women. Here too, an anesthetic is administered locally to prevent pain.

Electrodessication involves using an electric current to destroy the tissue. If you have a cardiac pacemaker, be sure to discuss it with your doctor. The high frequency of the electric current may disturb it.

A possible new alternative to the therapies for warts is a drug which comes in cream form and can be applied at home. It's called 5-fluorouracil and is sold under the brand names Fluoroplex® or Efudex®. It hasn't yet been approved by the Food and Drug Administration for use on warts, and there have been some reports that it can cause skin inflammation. Don't use it if you are pregnant.

Pregnancy and Warts

Birth control pills and pregnancy both stimulate the growth and spread of warts. In pregnancy, warts should be removed either by electrodessication or surgery. *Under no conditions should podophyllin be used,* since it is absorbed through the skin and can cause birth deformities or fetal death.

Researchers think that if warts aren't removed in pregnancy, the virus which causes them can be passed on to the infant at birth as it passes through the birth canal of an infected mother. This can cause warts in the larynx of the newborn. Laryngeal warts are potentially dangerous for an infant because they may spread into the bronchial tubes of the lungs, causing suffocation.

If a woman develops warts that obstruct the birth canal during pregnancy, a cesarean section will be performed.

Glossary

Alkaline Phosphatase—in diseases of the liver, the serum level of this substance rises. One of the tests used in diagnosing hepatitis measures the level of this substance.

Amoxicillin®—a penicillin-like medication for diseases caused by a variety of bacteria. Should not be taken by those allergic to penicillin.

Ampicillin—a penicillin-like medication, similar to amoxicillin in its anti-bacterial activity. Should not be taken by those allergic to penicillin.

Anoscope—a small speculum-like instrument that is inserted into the anus to examine the area. Should always be used to examine the anus of those engaging in anal receptive intercourse.

Antibiotic—a medication which has the power to inhibit the growth of or destroy specific microorganisms.

Antibody—a protein formed by the body to defend itself against a foreign substance.

Antigen—any substance which is capable of causing the formation of antibodies and is capable of reacting to them in some detectable manner. Used in laboratory tests for many diseases.

Asymptomatic—having a disease but not showing any symptoms.

Bicillin®—long-acting injectable penicillin used in the treatment of syphilis.

Bile—a fluid secreted by the liver.

Bilirubin—a bile pigment found in the plasma. When the liver is not functioning properly, it builds up in the body, coloring the urine brownish and giving the skin and whites of the eyes a yellowish appearance.

Bimanual pelvic examination—performed to check for pelvic inflammation and tenderness (for a complete description, refer to chapter on PID).

Biopsy—a bit of tissue is removed from the body and the cell types are examined under a microscope.

Cervix—passageway from a woman's vagina to her uterus (see illustrations on pp. 5–6).

Chlamydia—microorganism that causes a variety of diseases including nongonococcal urethritis and PID.

Congenital—refers to conditions that are present at birth.

Conjunctiva—the membrane that lines the eyelid and eyeball.

Conjunctivitis—an inflammation of the conjunctiva resulting in redness and a discharge.

Crotamiton—medication used for the treatment of scabies.

Cryotherapy—use of extreme cold to destroy body tissue. Used in the treatment of warts.

Culdocentesis—removing fluid from the uterine cavity. Performed in some cases of pelvic inflammatory disease to identify causative microorganisms.

Culture—growing microorganisms in an environment enriched with nutrients to encourage their reproduction. Used in many laboratory tests for disease.

Curet—a spoon-shaped instrument used for the removal of growths such as warts.

Cyst—(1) stage in the developmental life cycle of parasites during which they are enclosed inside a protective wall (2) a fluid-filled enlargement.

Cytotoxic agents—substances that have a toxic effect on cells. Used in the treatment of warts.

Darkfield examination—a microscopic test for syphilitic bacteria scraped from open sores.

Ectopic pregnancy—a pregnancy which does not develop in the uterus, usually located in the fallopian tube.

Electrodessication—using a high frequency electric current to dry up body tissue. Used in the treatment of warts.

Endometrium—the mucous membrane that lines the uterus.

Epididymis—tube-like structure on testes where sperm is stored (see illustrations on pp. 3–4).

Erythromycin—an alternative antibiotic for patients allergic to penicillin.

False positive blood test—positive reaction in syphilis serology testing that occurs in a small percentage of people who do not have the disease.

Flagyl®—brand name of the medication used for trichomoniasis and amebiasis. See metronidazole.

Fluorescent Treponemal Antibody (FTA)—blood test for syphilis.

Gram stain—special staining method used for identifying microorganisms on a slide under a microscope.

Granular erosions—small round masses of inflamed tissue.

Hemagglutination (HA) test—treponemal blood test for syphilis.

Herxheimer reaction—reaction that occurs within 12 hours after treatment for syphilis; caused by the destruction of treponemes in the body.

Immune serum globulin—serum containing large amounts of antibodies produced in response to antigens. It is given to people in contact with hepatitis to help prevent the disease.

Infestation—attack of the skin or organs of the body by parasites.

Keratitis—an inflammation of the cornea.

Kwell®—brand name for medication used in the treatment of scabies and crabs (see lindane).

Lactic dehydrogenase (LDH)—enzyme found in the blood and several organs. When the liver is diseased, as it is in hepatitis, the level of these enzymes will be elevated.

Laparoscopy—examination of the pelvic cavity with an instrument inserted through an incision in the navel.

Lindane—medication used in the treatment of crabs and scabies. Sold under the brand name Kwell®. Not recommended for use by pregnant women, infants and small children.

Metronidazole—medication effective against trichomoniasis, amebiasis and giardiasis. Since it has been shown to be carcinogenic in laboratory animals, unnecessary use of the drug should be avoided. The drug should not be taken by pregnant women in the first trimester.

Miconazole—anti-fungal medication used in the treatment of candidiasis.

Minocycline—a tetracycline-like antibiotic effective against a wide range of bacteria. Like tetracycline, the drug should not be taken by pregnant women, infants and children under the age of 8.

Monistat®—brand name for anti-fungal treatment used in candidiasis.

Mucous membrane—thin layer of tissue that lines the mouth, anus and genitals.

Mycoplasma—a broad label for several organisms in the urinary or genital tract which are responsible for some cases of nongonococcal urethritis (NGU).

Mycostatin®—brand name of anti-fungal medication used in the treatment of candidiasis.

Nystatin—anti-fungal medication used in the treatment of candidiasis.

Ophthalmia Neonatorum—extreme inflammation of the eye during the first ten days of life. Usually contracted during birth from infected discharge of the mother.

Pap smear—a staining procedure used mostly for detecting and diagnosing malignant and pre-malignant cells in the female genital tract. May also be used to aid in the diagnosis of herpes and trichomoniasis.

Pathogen—any disease-producing microorganism or material.

Penicillinase Producing Neisseria Gonorrhoeae (PPNG)—a strain of the gonococcus which is resistant to penicillin. Other medications, such as spectinomycin or tetracycline, are effective.

Perineum—the pelvic floor. The space between the anus and the urethra (see illustration on page 6).

Podophyllin—a chemical substance used in the treatment of warts (see cytotoxic agents).

Probenecid—medication used to increase the concentration of antibiotics in the blood. Given with penicillin in the treatment of gonorrhea.

Proctitis—inflammation of the rectum.

Prostate—a gland in the male which surrounds the urethra

and the neck of the bladder and contributes a secretion to the seminal fluid (see illustration on page 3).

Public Health Advisor—an individual who is specially trained in STD and works in public health clinics. The P.H.A. interviews patients with syphilis and traces their sexual contacts. S/he can usually answer questions and provide information about a variety of STDs.

Serofast—residual positive result in nontreponemal blood test for syphilis; remains positive even after adequate treatment.

Serum—the clear liquid component of blood.

Serum Glutamic Oxaloacetic Transaminase (SGOT)—enzyme found in the liver and other organs. When the liver is diseased, as in hepatitis, these enzymes leak into the blood. The level of SGOT in the blood provides useful information on the progress of hepatitis. In hepatitis, SGOT levels may be 10 to 100 times normal and remain elevated for a long time.

Serum Glutamic Pyruvic Transaminase (SGPT)—like the SGOT, the level of this enzyme in the blood will be elevated if the liver is diseased. In hepatitis, SGPT levels are higher than SGOT levels but should return to normal in two to three months.

Sitz Bath—a few inches of very hot water in a tub. Sitting in this with your feet propped up increases circulation to the affected area and helps healing.

Spectinomycin—injectable antibacterial medication used in the treatment of gonorrhea.

Steroids—hormone-like substances used for a wide range of symptoms and diseases. They should be used with caution.

Sulfonamide—a group of anti-bacterial drugs.

Tetracycline—broad spectrum antibiotic (see minocycline).

Thrush—candidiasis of the mucous membrane of the mouth of infants, often accompanied by fever and gastritis.

Titer—in syphilis serology tests, it is the quantity of a substance required to produce a reaction (see chapter on syphilis).

Toxin—a poisonous substance.

Treponemal blood tests—blood tests such as the FTA and HA used as confirmatory test in people suspected of having syphilis but who have no sign of the disease.

Treponeme—the pathogenic bacteria that causes syphilis.

Tzanck Test—examination of tissue from a lesion to diagnose the causative agent. Used in the diagnosis of herpes when there is a sore present.

Ureaplasma urealyticum—one of the organisms that commonly cause nongonococcal urethritis.

Urethra—the canal conveying urine from the bladder to the exterior of the body (see illustrations on pp. 3–6).

Urethritis—an inflammation of the urethra usually accompanied by a burning sensation upon urination and a discharge.

Venereal Disease Research Laboratory (VDRL)—common nontreponemal test used to detect syphilis.

Virus—minute infectious agent.

Wet Mount—test used in detecting causative organism for vaginitis. Specimen is taken from the vagina and placed on a slide with a drop of saline solution; it is examined under a microscope for presence of organisms.

Appendix A: How to Use a Speculum

Looking at one's own genitals ought to be as easy and natural as looking at one's own face. But for most women, it isn't.

Lots of us are just learning that our bodies really do belong to ourselves—to enjoy and to take care of. If we don't, we can't expect anybody else to.

The most challenging part of self-examination of the genitals is not really in what's to be done—that's all quite simple—but in learning to relax and take the time with your body. It can even turn out to be—dare we suggest it—fun.

Before we get down to specifics, here are some general points about knowing your body:

1. Make a conscious effort to note changes in your vaginal discharge during the course of a month. Sometimes there will be more, or it will be thicker, or change color. There is a normal pattern for each woman that occurs month after month. Departures from the pattern may indicate infection, as is sometimes the case, for example, with the three forms of vaginitis,* gonorrhea,* cervical herpes,* syphilis * and chlamydial infections.

If you are looking, you will notice your discharge when you wipe yourself after using the toilet, or on your underwear. For more careful examination, you can insert a tampon and then remove it, or a finger or use the speculum, which we'll describe in a minute.

2. Become familiar with your perineum—that whole area between your urethra and anus. Check out the various orifices and other features against the illustration on page 6. If you're used to seeing it in health, it'll be easy to spot a problem—a wart, a sore or a rash—should it occur. It's easiest to look at the perineum with the aid of a small mirror.
3. Let your fingers do the walking! Take a long tour, feeling the walls of the vagina and then all the way up to the cervix. If you have a diaphragm, you've been here many times before, but you may never have taken careful notice. You should be able to feel the os, the opening from the uterus into the vagina at the tip of the cervix. If you know how the vaginal tract usually feels, you'll know when something is wrong.

Using a Speculum

The speculum makes it possible for you to actually *see* inside the vagina and right up to the cervix. It's a handy little plastic instrument which costs little or nothing. Ask your doctor for one, or ask your local feminist health organization where you can get one, or contact a medical supply company.

To do the examination, you need a comfortable spot where you can sprawl on your back if you want to. You'll also need a strong beam of light directed between your legs; a rubberneck lamp would be ideal. And a hand-held mirror.

And the speculum. At first, it's going to look odd to you. Give yourself time to get acquainted with it: Open and close the blades several times and find out how it locks. It's really quite simple once you get the knack. Refer to the how-to illustrations.

Now, to insert it, you'll either want to lie on your back or sit up, legs apart and knees drawn up. Try using some pillows, under your head and under your hips. You slip the speculum in sideways; if it doesn't slip in easily, put some sterile lubricating jelly on the tip. When it's all the way in, turn it so the handle points up. Now lock it in an open position so that your hands are free to adjust the light and the mirror.

You should be able to see the cervix clearly. It's quite amazing the first time. The opening at the tip of the cervix is the os. There will probably also be a certain amount of discharge around the cervix.

Changes in the appearance of the cervix are often the first indication of several diseases in women. If you can detect change at the cervix, you may be able to prevent the spread of several serious infections. Growths, sores, swelling, unusual coloration of the cervix and changes in the amount, color and odor of the secretions around the cervix—all these are excellent reasons to consult a doctor.

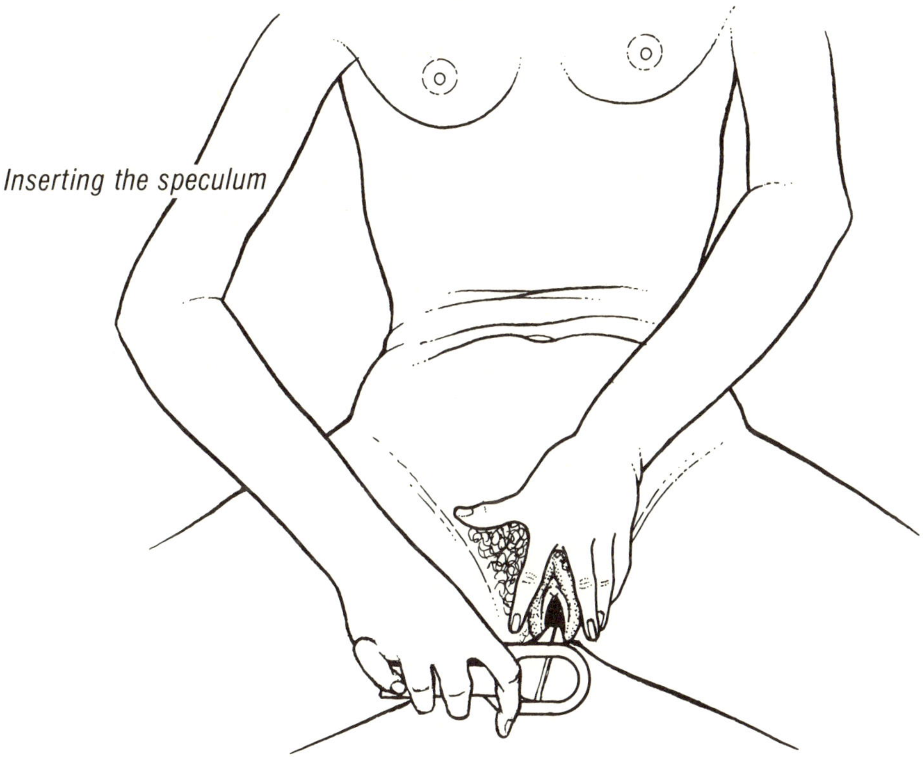
Inserting the speculum

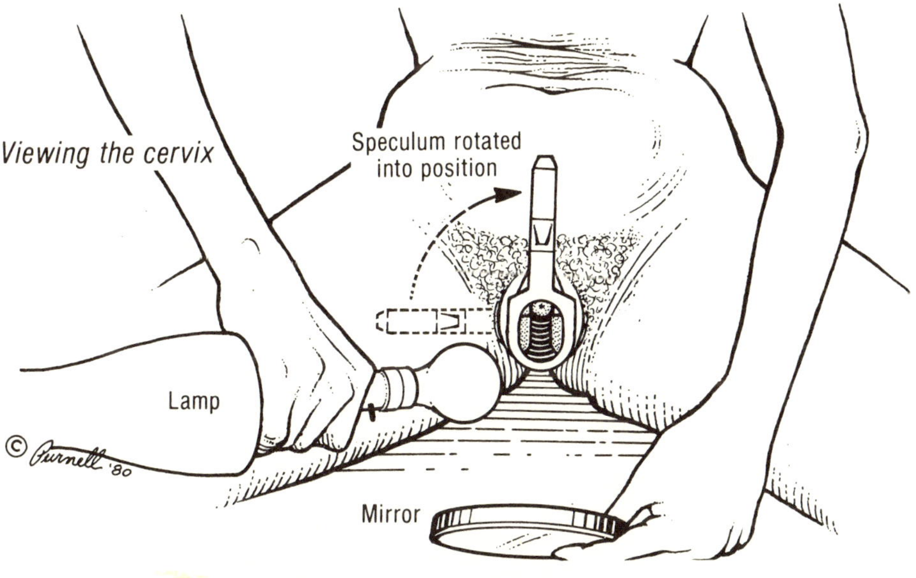
Viewing the cervix
Speculum rotated
into position
Lamp
Mirror
© Purnell '80

Appendix B: How to Find Proper Testing and Treatment

UNLESS YOU'RE WEALTHY, or lucky, it's often difficult to find health care providers whom you are completely satisfied with. This is even more of a challenge with sexually transmissible diseases, since many doctors don't feel knowledgeable or comfortable with respect to them.

There are several factors that will play a role in determining what sort of facility is the best for you: the geographic location and the size of the community you live in; your sex; your sexual preferences; your pocketbook; your symptoms; and your personality. Here's some information which may make your decisions easier.

The Public Health Clinics

They're free, almost always (and when not, it's only a nominal charge). There are thousands of them all over the country. They are all equipped to:

—do smears and cultures for gonorrhea, and treat it
—do darkfield examinations and blood tests for syphilis, and treat it
—diagnose and treat PID

—offer the services of a Public Health Advisor, who is specially trained to answer questions about STD, even over the telephone.

In addition, some of the larger urban clinics offer:

—treatment for NGU
—diagnosis of the forms of vaginitis, and treatment or a prescription for medication
—diagnosis of herpes
—diagnosis of crabs and scabies.

The National VD Hotline (1-800-227-8922) can direct you to the nearest health facility and answer any questions you may have. The call is free. None of the public clinics test or treat hepatitis, cystitis or the enteric STDs. With these you have the choice of going to a doctor's office or to a hospital outpatient clinic.

The public health clinics are highly experienced in dealing with gonorrhea and syphilis. But individual clinics can vary widely in their experience with other STDs and in the quality of patient care. You can determine the range of their services, their hours and their charges if any with a phone call. But to determine the quality of patient care, you'll probably have to make a visit or ask a friend who's been there.

Outside of the urban centers, a public health clinic may offer only minimal services. It will refer you to a private physician or a hospital clinic if your symptoms indicate a disease it doesn't treat. Doctors are required to treat any information you give them as confidential and it is important that you trust your doctor to do this so that you can supply him/her with all the background information necessary to diagnose a disease.

Choosing a Doctor

A doctor doesn't have to be a specialist to treat STD. What is important is that s/he sees a large number of people with these diseases and has experience and up-to-date information on their treatment and management.

STD is an area of medicine that is changing as the incidence of the diseases increases. Advances and new discoveries are constantly being made. And as with everything else, the more someone does something, the better s/he gets at it. There is no substitute for clinical experience.

Also, STDs that are prevalent in some communities, aren't in others. Doctors seeing large numbers of STD patients will be aware of what to look for and what particular diseases are common in their communities.

The following is not an ironclad law, but it does generally hold true: Women are often more comfortable with women doctors and gay men are more comfortable with gay doctors. It tends to be easier to tell people of like sex and sexual preferences about yourself, including your sexual behavior, your symptoms and your worries.

This is not to say that a male doctor can't be excellent and understanding to women, or that a heterosexual doctor is not sympathetic to gays. But if you are uncomfortable with your doctor, it's time to shop around for another one.

• Women can call the National Organization for Women (N.O.W.) headquarters, located in Washington, D.C., to get the location of the nearest N.O.W. office. It may have a listing of local women doctors, or members may refer you to doctors they have used and liked.

Or you can call the National Women's Health Network in Washington, D.C. They can direct you to the feminist health clinic nearest to you. While most feminist clinics are not equipped to deal with a wide range of STDs, you will certainly be able to speak with a sympathetic professional who will put you on the right track.

There is a Women's Medical Association (the female counterpart to the A.M.A.) in every state. You can call them and get a list of women doctors who are members.

• Gay men in many major cities have organized volunteer clinics which offer information, testing and even treatment for some of the STDs. They'll also refer you to sympathetic doctors. Or you can call your local Gay Switchboard for information. The best way, of course, to find a good doctor is usually through the recommendations of friends.

If you aren't in a major city or don't have access to the above routes call the National VD Hotline (1-800-227-8922)—it's free. Or you might invest in a copy of the *Gayellow Pages* for your area ($1.95, Renaissance House, Box 292, Village Station, N.Y., 10014/ tel. (212) 929-7720). It'll list the gay health facility nearest you or where to go for information.

• A very good general reference for anyone who is looking for a doctor is the *State Medical Directory*. It lists all M.D.s who are licensed to practice in the state, tells you where and when they got their education, what their specialty is and whether they are affiliated with a hospital. It also lists hospitals city by city, their staff physicians and departments. Your local library will probably have a copy at the reference desk.

Of course, if you are having sudden and acute pains, rush straight to your nearest hospital emergency room. But *if you are a sexually active person, you should probably look for a doctor before you get symptoms of a particular STD.* It is very reassuring to know a doctor who knows you and your history, who you can see when you need to, and can even call up from time to time.

The choice of a doctor is very personal. Until you find

someone whom you feel comfortable with, you should feel absolutely free to shop around, talk to everyone you know, inquire about prices and, finally, talk at length with a doctor at your first appointment.

Some of the things you should expect from a doctor are:

- an explanation of any tests ordered, including prices and possible risks.
- explanations of test results—ask for the exact values and get the doctor to tell you what the normal range is. If a culture is done, you'll be calling to ask for the results. If any results are positive, expect medical attention from your doctor until the results return to normal.
- an explanation of any diagnosis the doctor makes—ask about the sickness: Is it catching or will it spread? How could it have been prevented? What will the course of the illness be? How long does it usually take to recover? What signs of relapse should you watch for?
- detailed information about any drug prescribed. Ask about possible side effects; about alternative drugs and alternative drug-free therapy. Make sure you understand how and when and for how long to take a drug; whether you should avoid any foods, activities or other medicines while taking it; what you should do if you miss a pill. *Ask the doctor to prescribe drugs by their generic names.* You can save money.

The Physicians' Desk Reference (PDR) is a book that contains all the information you would want to know about most prescription drugs. This includes: how the drug works; which diseases it's prescribed for; possible side effects; safety of the drug in pregnancy; warnings about hazards posed by the drug. It's available at the reference desk of most public libraries or can be purchased for about $15. If you have trouble with the technical language, you can refer to a medical dictionary.

Doing Your Part

This is a two-way street. If you've found a good doctor treat him or her well. Above all be truthful and honest. Speaking out honestly about your sexuality is a critical component of your health care, particularly with STDs. It's essential that the doctor know which orifices should be examined. If you are nervous about the confidentiality of the information, discuss this too with your doctor. A sympathetic doctor can word diagnoses on official records—such as company insurance forms—so that there is no embarrassment.

Asking questions serves at least two important purposes: It lets a doctor know you're interested, and it gives you a chance to learn more about your own body and how your doctor operates. It's a good idea to write questions down before you go. Reading up about an illness you have or might have will make it easier for you to grasp what the doctor says.

Once you've got a good doctor, let the relationship grow. Make sure your doctor knows you like and trust him/her. It's a definite advantage to have one doctor who knows you and treats you over a long period of time.

Appendix C: How Not to Use this Book: Prevention

YOU KNOW WHAT Smokey the Bear always says! Of course, we're not suggesting that STD can be completely eliminated, but we *can* limit it to short and infrequent outbursts and keep it from raging out of control.

There may come a day when you can line up at your local clinic for immunization inoculations against, say, gonorrhea or herpes, but that is certainly a long way off. Until then, survival involves taking responsibility for stopping STD at your own doorstep.

The medical literature on prevention is awfully cynical about getting people to do something about it themselves. But we think, if you are reading this book, you've already made a first step. So we'd like to lay it on the line without mincing words: *Nothing will work unless you make it work.*

And after all, isn't it worth it? Sex is an important part of our lives. We derive a great deal of pleasure from it and, possibly, we could derive more if we take the time and effort to think our way through to an intelligent attitude about our sexual relations and our own body. If you think planning might take some of the fun out of "spontaneous" sex, just consider how much fun STD can take out of it.

One night stands—and encounters of even briefer duration—are the nemesis of VD control programs, since a disease can be transmitted far and wide between people who don't even know each other's names and phone numbers. We aren't advocating any particular sexual practices; the length of an encounter doesn't necessarily say anything about its quality. But we do think that we owe it to each other—for our psychological as well as physical well-being—to be more open and honest with each other.

The kind of openness we are talking about begins at home with your own body. It's possible—and important—to be as familiar with your genitalia as you are with your face. First of all, there is absolutely nothing wrong with it, although many of us have been brought up to think there is. And second of all, there are many illnesses which you can detect at an early stage by being sensitive to yourself; if you do, you'll be able to treat them before they get serious and you won't go around unknowingly transmitting them to others.

Since men handle their penis every day, the above idea is probably not quite so foreign to them as it is to many women, whose sexual organs are more difficult to see. One of the major tenets of the women's movement has been that sexual equality and good health must rest on self-knowledge. The mechanics of the foray into the unknown are described in Appendix A.

For both men and women, the subject of rectal intercourse is often even more shrouded with shame and secrecy than other sexual activities. There's no reason for this. Rectal intercourse is a legitimate form of sexual activity which —if accompanied by good personal hygiene—is just as safe as other forms of sex. Some people like it, others don't. (We must caution, however, that the insertion of other objects into the anus is frequently hazardous.)

The other part of the open equation is communication between sex partners. No matter how fleeting an encounter is, it demands a certain amount of trust. It's possible and important to put that trust on firm ground by making the circumstances as reassuring as possible. That means, at the very least, that you are able to trade names and phone numbers with sex partners so that you can notify each other in case a problem does arise.

Even where sexual encounters are anonymous, you can improve your chances of avoiding disease by asking for screening facilities. In several cities, the gay community has succeeded in having STD screening in the bath houses. Organized political action could go a long way toward improving medical attention to STD. While the gay community has been most successful, any group willing to recognize the need for improved care—women, for example, or educators—can influence the way the government spends its VD control funds.

Preventive Techniques

None of them perform miracles, but if they are used consistently and carefully, and in combination with a caring attitude toward yourself and your sex partners, you will be able to avoid most of the trouble of STD.

SELECTIVITY Celibacy is extreme and, if you are reading this book, we assume you're not really interested. But what about good old common sense? That means choosing only those partners whom you are fairly sure of or refraining from some kinds of activity in doubtful situations. The fewer people you are with and the fewer orifices entered, naturally, the fewer chances of contracting a disease.

MECHANICAL BARRIERS CONDOMS are great, inexpensive, easy to buy and portable. Unfortunately they've become less popular ever since the "miracle" contraceptives came on the market in the '60s. Nevertheless, condoms remain the single most effective way of preventing sexually transmitted disease as well as unwanted babies.

We think there's a renaissance on the way for condoms. We've noticed large, colorful displays lately in our neighborhood drugstores, offering a variety of brands from $2.50 per dozen and up. The more expensive ones are usually kept behind the counter; lambskins can go as high as $15 for twelve. It's a matter of personal taste and pocketbook, but they're all about equally efficient. It's worth buying several brands and trying them out; you can get them in different colors and textures.

DIAPHRAGMS are effective as barriers against disease, mostly because of the contraceptive cream or jelly that's used with them. Any bacteria traveling up the vaginal canal will most likely be stopped dead at the diaphragm. But, obviously, this will not protect the anus, the mouth or the anterior part of the vagina.

CONTRACEPTIVE CREAMS, JELLIES AND TABLETS are proven effective against gonorrhea, syphilis, candidiasis and trichomoniasis. If you use the pill or the IUD for contraception, it's wise to use one of these to prevent sexually transmissible disease.

Because, *the pill and the IUD are totally ineffective in preventing disease.*

What's more, *the pill sometimes promotes the growth of both gonorrhea and anogenital warts, as well as certain kinds of vaginitis,* by altering the environment of the vagina.

And *the IUD aids the spread of the gonococcal bacteria* into the fallopian tubes, where it can cause real damage.

SYSTEMIC PREVENTION The idea is great. Wouldn't it be nice if you could take a pill and then be completely free of worries about sexually transmissible disease? Well, there is no such pill and probably never will be because of the great variety of pathogens involved in STD.

There is selective chemical prevention, however, an antibiotic regimen which reduces the chances of gonorrhea and syphilis infection (and, if it's tetracycline, NGU also). This is definitely a possibility for those people who are constantly exposed to gonorrhea and syphilis. But it won't work if the gonorrhea and syphilis pathogens are resistant and, we repeat, it won't work for hepatitis, herpes and all the other STDs. Individuals often develop an allergic response to the medication. On a broader scale, widespread use will encourage the development of more resistant strains of the bacteria.

You and your doctor must balance the pros and cons, considering your own particular circumstances when taking this step.

GENERAL CLEANLINESS Bacteria, virus, fungi, parasites, they're all so tiny they're easy to forget about, especially when you're having a good time. Don't. Be aware that pathogens can live for hours, not only on the body, but on sheets, towels and clothing.

No need to be paranoid; just remember that washing with soap and water helps keep the spread of disease under control. Especially when a penis is inserted into the anus, it should be washed before insertion into any other orifice. If you're using a lubricant, make sure it's one of the water-based ones that can be washed away (like K-Y Jelly ®). An uncircumcised penis should be washed very carefully. Urination after intercourse, by both men and women, keeps down the growth of bacteria and other pathogens.

Routine douching for women is not recommended. There are exceptions (see chapter on vaginitis). Although some douching formulas are antibiotic, the pressure of the water entering the vaginal canal can push bacteria up the passageway and through the cervical os to the uterus, where they can ascend into the fallopian tubes and do serious damage.

PERSONAL HEALTH CARE It goes almost without saying that the healthier you are, the more successful your body will be in defending itself from infection. Nobody is invulnerable, but good nutrition, exercise and sufficient rest can go a long way toward lessening your chances of becoming ill, and shorten the duration of any condition you might contract.

The choice of a doctor who is right for you is terribly important for your health. You should be able to call for advice, speak freely and trust what your doctor says and does. We go into more detail about your choice of a doctor in Appendix B.

No doctor can do the job alone. If you are diagnosed for an STD, find out about it. Understand the medication you are taking. And make sure you are taking it correctly. If you have any doubts or questions, ask your doctor or pharmacist.

Finally, to repeat the constant refrain of this book: *Prevent reinfection from sexual partners* by encouraging them to attend to their health also.

Index

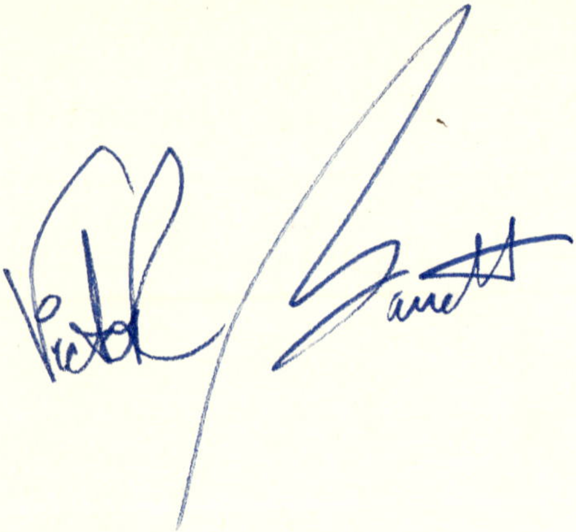